Hypnosis and Hypnotherapy

Hypnosis and Hypnotherapy

Volume 2: Applications in Psychotherapy and Medicine

Deirdre Barrett, Editor

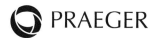 PRAEGER

AN IMPRINT OF ABC-CLIO, LLC
Santa Barbara, California • Denver, Colorado • Oxford, England

Library of Congress Cataloging-in-Publication Data

Hypnosis and hypnotherapy / Deirdre Barrett, editor.
    p. ; cm.
  Includes bibliographical references and index.
  ISBN 978-0-313-35632-2 (hard copy : alk. paper) — ISBN 978-0-313-
35633-9 (ebook) — ISBN 978-0-313-35634-6 (vol. 1 hard copy : alk.
paper) — ISBN 978-0-313-35635-3 (vol. 1 ebook) — ISBN 978-0-313-
35636-0 (vol. 2 hard copy : alk. paper) — ISBN 978-0-313-35637-7 (vol.
2 ebook)
  1. Hypnotism. 2. Hypnotism—Therapeutic use. I. Barrett,
Deirdre.
  [DNLM: 1. Hypnosis—methods. 2. Mental Disorders—therapy. WM 415
H9961 2010]
  RC495.H963   2010
  615.8′512—dc22   2010015824

ISBN: 978-0-313-35632-2
EISBN: 978-0-313-35633-9

14 13 12 11 10   1 2 3 4 5

This book is also available on the World Wide Web as an eBook.
Visit www.abc-clio.com for details.

Praeger
An Imprint of ABC-CLIO, LLC

ABC-CLIO, LLC
130 Cremona Drive, P.O. Box 1911
Santa Barbara, California 93116-1911

This book is printed on acid-free paper ∞

Manufactured in the United States of America

Contents

Acknowledgments

I would like to thank Debbie Carvalko from Praeger Publishers for her advocacy of this project, and for her advice, organization, and review of these volumes. I would also like to thank the book's advisory board: Arreed Barabasz, PhD, EdD; Elvira Lang, MD; Steve Lynn, PhD; and David Spiegel, MD, for their help in identifying topics to be covered and advice on the best authors to cover them.

Finally, I want to acknowledge the professional hypnosis societies that introduced me to the members of the advisory board and to most of the chapter authors. These organizations taught me much of the hypnosis I've learned since my basic graduate school training, as they have for many of the chapter authors. They provide forums in which advances in hypnosis are shared in a timely manner among practitioners. The first two societies listed here publish academic journals in which much of the research and clinical techniques summarized in these volumes has appeared. All five conduct stimulating conferences with research presentations and workshops—for students as well as practicing professionals. All maintain referral lists from which potential clients can locate skilled hypnotherapists in their geographic area. They constitute a rich resource for readers wishing to pursue more learning about hypnosis.

The Society for Clinical and Experimental Hypnosis
SCEH Executive Office
P.O. Box 252
Southborough, MA 01772
Tel: 508-598-5553
Fax: 866-397-1839
Email: info@sceh.us
Publishes *International Journal of Clinical and Experimental Hypnosis*

American Society of Clinical Hypnosis
140 N. Bloomingdale Rd.
Bloomingdale, IL 60108
Telephone: 630-980-4740
Fax: 630-351-8490
Email: info@asch.net
Publishes *American Journal of Clinical Hypnosis*

Society of Psychological Hypnosis
Division 30–American Psychological Association
APA Division 30 Membership
1400 N. La Salle, Unit 3-S
Chicago, IL 60610
http://www.apa.org/divisions/div30/homepage.html

European Society for Hypnosis
ESH Central Office
Inspiration House
Redbrook Grove
Sheffield, S20 6RR
United Kingdom
Telephone : +44 11 4248 8917
Fax : +44 11 4247 4627
E-mail : mail@esh-hypnosis.eu
http://www.esh-hypnosis.eu/index.php?folder_id=14&file_id=0

International Society for Hypnosis
http://www.ish-web.org/page.php

Introduction

Deirdre Barrett

Hypnosis is named for the Greek god of sleep though, even in ancient times, few thought of it as literal sleep—this was simply the best analogy for an altered state so far from waking cognition and behavior. Western medicine first called the phenomena "mesmerism" after Franz Mesmer, who conducted group trance inductions in eighteenth-century Europe. Mesmer attracted attention for his flamboyant style and his cures of hysteria that eluded other physicians of the time. Of course, Mesmer did not invent hypnosis, he merely rediscovered techniques that had been practiced around the world since the dawn of history. A fourth-century BCE Egyptian demotic papyrus from Thebes describes a boy being induced into a healing trance by eye fixation on a lighted lamp.[1] Third-century BCE Greek temples in Epidaurus and Kos, dedicated to the god Asclepius—whose snake-entwined staff is now our modern medical symbol, the caduceus—used hypnotic-like incubation rituals to produce their dramatic cures.[2] Mesmer's contribution was that he reminded the Western world of this marvelous therapy. Young doctors flocked to him to study, but the medical establishment was no friendlier to alternative medicine then than now. Mesmer was exiled from medical practice, but therapists and the general public have remained fascinated with hypnosis ever since.

In recent years, we have been able to understand hypnosis much better than Mesmer did with his eighteenth-century versions of magnetic and electrical fields of the body. Indeed we are able to see what real changes in brain activity occur during the process, but also a wealth of modern cognitive, linguistic, and personality research help explain it. *Hypnosis and Hypnotherapy* brings together the latest research on the nature of hypnosis and studies of what it can accomplish in treatment. Volume 1 addresses the question of what hypnosis is: the cognitions, brain activity, and personality traits that characterize it, as well as cultural beliefs about hypnosis. In Chapter 1, Robert Kunzendorf describes how cognitive processing differs during hypnosis from usual waking modes. He characterizes the core change as "the deactivation of self-conscious source monitoring." This lack of awareness of the self as the origin of many perceptions during hypnosis leads to experiencing imagery as hallucinations and to alterations of memory processing including dissociation, amnesia, and hypermnesia. Kunzendorf explains how these changes can sometimes enable hypnosis to recover repressed memories but also increase the possibility of creating false ones.

The most common misconception in hypnosis lore is the notion that trance, hallucinatory imagery, the will to carry out suggestions—indeed all the phenomena of hypnosis—emanate from the hypnotist. In fact, it is the subject who produces these. In Chapter 2, I examine personality traits associated with the ability to enter hypnotic trance. Very few people are totally unhypnotizable, but the number able to experience the deepest hypnotic phenomena—eyes open hallucinations, negative hallucinations (failing to perceive something that is right in front of one), suggested amnesia and analgesia sufficient for surgery—is similarly small. Hypnotizability is not a present/absent dichotomy but a continuum. Many traits were historically hypothesized to determine hypnotizability such as hysteric personality, passivity, "weak will," and "need to please," but these actually bear little or no correlation when subjected to modern research analyses. This chapter summarizes the cluster of traits that do predict response to hypnotic induction. All of the interview and test questions that correlate highly concern hypnotic-like experiences of everyday life vividness of imagery, propensity to daydream, and the ability to block out real sensory stimuli. I also present a distinction between two types of high hypnotizables—one of whom has more of a propensity toward vivid, hallucinatory imagery, and the other toward dissociative, amnestic separation of memory. The first group "fantasizers" tend to have a history of parents who read them much fiction and encouraged fantasy play, while the second group "dissociaters" have a history of trauma or isolation during which they learned amnestic defenses.

In Chapter 3, David Spiegel, Matthew White, and Lynn Waelde review the effects of hypnosis on physiologic functions. Past studies have found that induction of the hypnotic state reduces sympathetic nervous system activity and increases parasympathetic activity, as measured by the low frequency/high frequency ratio in spectral analysis of heart rate, and by increases in vagal tone. Both of these changes are associated with the ability to self-soothe. Hypnosis has also been found to affect the secretion of cortisol and prolactin and to modulate other neural and endocrine components of the stress response. The authors then describe recent brain imaging of hypnosis at their lab and other research facilities. The most consistent changes are found in the frontal attentional systems. Spiegel, White, and Waelde explain why these often track with the alterations of autonomic tone noted in the peripheral studies of hypnosis. They describe how hypnosis is associated with changes in the executive attention function of the anterior cingulate gyrus and involves "activation" rather than "arousal" in neurological terms—and dopaminergic rather than noradrenergic in biochemical ones. This type of activation promotes "chunking," or reducing the number of parallel systems, and indicates an inner rather than outer focus. Spiegel, White, and Waelde compare brain imaging findings in hypnosis with those associated with mindfulness meditation and discuss the physiological similarity of states produced by the two techniques. Finally, they discuss shifts in brain activity associated with particular hypnotic phenomena such as alterations of pain perception and with the lessened sense of self-agency during hypnosis that was characterized as essential in Chapter 1.

In Chapter 4, Melvin Gravitz describes forensic hypnosis—the role it has played in police investigation and the court system. Views of hypnosis have swung from touting hypnosis as a truth serum to seeing it as inherently invalidating witness testimony. Gravitz reviews the precedents and opinions at all levels, up to and including the U.S. Supreme Court, and offers his own balanced view of appropriate uses and safeguards. He discusses how the hypnotic alterations of memory discussed in Chapters 1 and 3, and the hypnotic-associated personality traits dealt with in Chapter 2, manifest specifically during criminal witness proceedings. Next, in Chapter 5, I discuss the depiction of hypnosis in art and media—film, television, theater, music, and cartoons. These depictions emphasize behavioral control rather than rich alterations of subjective experience. Most films cast hypnosis in a dark light—as a tool for seduction or murder. When hypnosis is portrayed positively, it is often either as a truth serum—similar to the overly optimistic court opinions discussed in Chapter 4 (in fact, these often appear in courtroom dramas) or as endowing subjects with impossible psychological, mental, or athletic abilities. The chapter concludes with a discussion of how more realistic depictions of hypnosis in media might be encouraged.

In Chapter 6, Stanley Krippner and Jürgen Kremer discuss hypnotic-like practices in shamanism and folk medium traditions with illustrative examples from various North American tribes, Balinese folk customs, contemporary Sámi (indigenous Scandinavian) practices and African-Brazilian mediumship. They describe the many similarities in these societies' inductions and Western hypnosis, including verbal inductions and suggestion, sleep analogies, and heavy reliance on imagery and storytelling (the latter being characteristic mostly of Ericksonian hypnosis to be described in Volume 2, Chapter 1, rather than of all Western hypnosis). Krippner and Kremer also contrast trance-induction practices that are common in the indigenous cultures but not in Western hypnosis including chanting, percussion, dance or other ritualistic movement, and the burning of incense. They note a fundamental difference in the two types of indigenous practices of shamanism versus mediumship. Shamans are usually aware of everything that occurs while they converse with spirits, even when a spirit "speaks through" them, whereas mediums claim to lose awareness once they incorporate a spirit, and purport to remember little about the experience once the spirit departs. This distinction is similar to the two types of high hypnotizables—fantasizers and dissociaters—described in Chapter 2. Krippner and Kremer describe how these cultures foster fantasy proneness and train dissociation to some degree, but that there also seem to be significant "demand characteristics" to produce the culturally sanctioned behavior. Krippner has also researched individual variables of subjects within these cultures, finding some of the same characteristics associated with improvement by Western psychotherapy such as "willingness to change one's behavior" predict beneficial outcome to treatment with shaman or medium.

In Chapter 7, Steve Eichel describes the responses of the main lay hypnosis credentialing groups (those not associated with the mental health professionals, dentistry or medicine, but purporting to represent the "profession" of hypnosis) to applications for credentialing from a distinctly unqualified practitioner . . . his pet cat Zoe. Eichel uses the humorous ploy of getting Zoe certified with applications listing study at ImaCat U and hefty licensing fees to point out what's wrong with the concept of commercial "credentialing" groups unaffiliated with state licensing or university certification. Eichel goes on to describe why it is important to have clinicians trained in the underlying disorders that they are treating before applying hypnosis to them.

Finally, in Chapter 8, Ian Wickramasekera describes in more detail how this training should be conducted. He reviews the history of how hypnosis has been taught—in Western psychotherapy and medicine, but also in the indigenous cultures covered in Chapter 6, ending with a description of the modern training guidelines established by the American Society of Clinical Hypnosis. Wickramasekera discusses how it is possible to draw together the best elements of each of these different pedagogical traditions into a training program for teaching hypnosis either within a university setting or a postgraduate certificate program.

Volume 2 addresses the clinical applications of hypnosis in psychotherapy and medicine. In the term *hypnotherapy*, the second half of the term is as important as the first. Except for some generalized effects on relaxation and stress reduction, it is not the state of hypnosis itself that affects change, but rather the images and suggestions that are utilized while in the hypnotic state. Because hypnosis bypasses the conscious mind's habits and resistances, it is often quicker than other forms of therapy, and its benefits may appear more dramatically. However, the reputed dangers of hypnotherapy are really those of all therapy: first, that an overzealous therapist may push the patient to face what has been walled off for good reason before new strengths are in place; and second, that the therapist will abuse his or her position of persuasion. People come to hypnotherapy with similar complaints and hopes to those they bring to any treatment for physical or psychological problems. Despite the added role of hypnotizability, most of the same factors determine the outcome: the skill of the therapist, the patient's motivation to drop old patterns, the rapport between patient and therapist, and how supportive family and friends are of change.

Volume 2 begins by introducing the different branches of hypnotic psychotherapy. In Chapter 1, Stephen Lankton describes Ericksonian hypnotherapy—the approach derived from the body of writing, training, and lectures of the late Milton Erickson. Ericksonian techniques include designing individualized inductions in the client's distinctive language, incorporating the client's metaphors for their disorders into the suggestions for change and using indirect suggestion—which is ambiguous, vague, and more permissive—to avoid provoking resistance. In Chapter 2, Arreed Barabasz traces the history of psychodynamic and ego psychology applications to hypnosis and then describes in more detail modern ego state hypnotherapy. Ego state theory posits that people's personalities are separated into various segments. Unique entities serve different purposes. Ego states often start as defensive coping mechanisms and develop into compartmentalized sections of the personality, but they may also be created by a single incident of trauma. Ego states maintain their own memories and communicate with other ego states to a greater or lesser degree. Unlike alters in multiple personalities, ego states are a part of normal personalities. Conflicts among states take up considerable energy, often forcing the individual into withdrawn, defensive postures. Hypnosis can facilitate communication between ego states, allow memories associated with one to become available to the whole person, and teach people to shift states more consciously and adaptively.

Chapter 3 continues the discussion of psychodynamic uses of hypnosis, with my summary of the research and clinical work on hypnotic dreams and the variety of ways of combining hypnosis and dreamwork for the mutual enhancement of each. One can use hypnotic suggestions that a person will experience a dream in the trance state—either as an open-ended suggestion or with the suggestion that they dream about a certain topic—and these "hypnotic dreams" have been found to be similar enough to nocturnal dreams to be worked with using many of the same techniques usually applied to nocturnal dreams. One can also work with previous nocturnal dreams during a hypnotic trance in ways parallel to Jung's "active imagination" techniques to continue, elaborate on, or explore the meaning of the dream. Research has also found that hypnotic suggestions can be used to influence future nocturnal dream content, and that hypnotic suggestions can increase the frequency of laboratory-verified lucid dreams. Hypnotic suggestion can also be used simply to increase nocturnal dream recall.

In Chapter 4, Michael Yapko discusses the newest branch of hypnotherapy—cognitive behavioral—and especially its use in treating depression. He describes how the classic conceptualization of hypnosis as "believed-in imagination" is consistent with modern cognitive behavioral theory. Hypnosis can serve as a means of absorbing people in new ways of thinking about their subjective experience and as a method of replacing automatic negative thoughts with positive beliefs and expectancies. It can foster skill acquisition, breaking old associations and instilling new ones. Yapko reviews the growing body of research on the effectiveness of such techniques. Finally, because insomnia is such a common symptom of depression, he describes in detail how hypnosis can resolve insomnia by inducing relaxation and interrupting the ruminations that interfere with sleep.

The remainder of the volume addresses applications of hypnosis to medical problems. In Chapter 5, Nicole Flory and Elvira Lang review the use of hypnosis for analgesia from nineteenth-century surgery prior to the discovery of ether up to modern times. The authors describe how surgery has evolved from more traditional large-incision techniques toward the insertion of surgical instruments through tiny skin openings under the guidance of X-rays, ultrasound, magnet resonance imaging (MRI), and endoscopes. They then review in detail their own carefully controlled research on utilizing hypnosis to alleviate pain, anxiety, and other distress associated with surgery in the new interventional radiological settings. Despite previous speculation by others that it would add excessive costs or time to the procedures, the authors found that teaching hypnosis-naive patients techniques on the operating table shortened procedures by decreasing patient interference and decreased costs by lowering subsequent complication rates. In addition to reducing the main target symptoms of pain and anxiety, hypnotic interventions kept patients' blood pressure and heart rate more stable. Flory and Lang conclude that hypnotic techniques can be safely and effectively integrated into high-tech medical environments.

In Chapter 6, Kent Cadegan and Krishna Kumar review studies on using hypnosis to treat smoking, alcoholism, and drug abuse. There is much more research on its use for smoking cessation than for any other addictive disorder. They report that results are encouraging even for two-session hypnotic smoking cessation treatment, but that there is no evidence for the efficacy of the one-session approach, though clinically, this is frequently practiced. Efficacy of hypnotherapy is less rigorously documented for other addictions, though there is growing interest in its use. Research on hypnosis to aid sobriety in alcoholics has found positive effects, but with small sample sizes and only short-term follow-up. There is less data yet on hypnotic interventions in drug addiction. In one recent study, veterans at an outpatient substance abuse treatment center benefitted from training in self-hypnosis, with a very strong main effect for practice—the more regularly they practiced their self-hypnotic suggestions, the likelier they were to remain abstinent. Cadegan and Kumar predict that, with more research like this, it will eventually become possible to say to a potential client that hypnosis can help them control their addiction if they have certain characteristics (e.g., hypnotizability, motivation to quit, and availability of social support), and if they are willing to practice (with specification about the nature and amount of practice).

Finally, in Chapter 7, Nicholas A. Covino, Jessica Wexler, and Kevin Miller briefly review the research on hypnotic pain control, already described in Chapter 6 as establishing a clear efficacy for hypnosis in that area. They then review the research on hypnosis in other health related areas, such as insomnia, asthma, bulimia, and a number of more function gastrointestinal disorders such as hypermotility (leading to cramps and chronic diarrhea) and hyperemesis (uncontrolled vomiting, usually due either to cancer chemotherapy or as a complication of pregnancy). They conclude that results on all these disorders are clearly positive but need more research. They emphasize the point—which is true of both application of hypnosis to psychotherapy discussed earlier in this volume and to its role in medicine—that there is great promise for its use with many illnesses and conditions. However, for hypnosis to be better accepted, it is imperative that researchers in the field update older studies with ones that pay more attention to current norms of "empirically validated treatments" and integrate promising strategies from related research such as the mindfulness meditation discussed in Volume 1, Chapter 3. Then this powerful technique will begin to be applied to many disorders in a way that it is currently only utilized routinely for pain control, anxiety, and smoking cessation.

NOTES

1. Griffith, F. I. & Herbert Thompson (Eds.) (1974) *The Leyden Papyrus: An Egyptian Magical Book*. New York: Dover Publications.
2. Hart, Gerald (2000) *Asclepius: The God of Medicine*. London: Royal Society of Medicine Press.

Chapter 1

Ericksonian Approaches to Hypnosis and Therapy

Stephen R. Lankton

INTRODUCTION

The focus for this chapter is an approach to change based upon the life work of Milton Erickson, MD. This is often referred to as the Ericksonian Approach to hypnosis and therapy. It represents a distinctive and effective approach to psychotherapy and the use of hypnosis as an adjunct to psychotherapy (Zeig, 1982). Dr. Erickson's approach can be distinguished by differences between his selection and use of therapeutic content and in handling of the process of change in psychotherapy. Ironically, process and content distinctions are themselves sometimes blurred in Ericksonian approaches, and these points will be discussed.

HISTORY AND BACKGROUND

The Ericksonian Approach has been derived from the body of work, training, and lectures provided by Milton Erickson, MD (1901–1980). Erickson was generally acknowledged to be the world's leading practitioner of medical or clinical hypnosis. His name and his ideas have been used by many professionals to denote some aspect of their work. However, it is often unclear what specific aspect of their work merits that distinction. This presents a difficulty I will address later. Similarly, with the rise of a rash of nonprofessionals who refer to themselves as "certified hypnotherapists," even greater reference is made to their so-called "Ericksonian Hypnotherapy." As with other approaches to change, such as Gestalt therapy and cognitive behavior therapy, there is no formal body of control over the use of Erickson's name.

There is no universally accepted and established standard on how one interprets Erickson's practices or how one applies his approach in treatment. While this situation may lead to much misinformation, there are several scholarly works written by Erickson and about his work that preserve an accurate record of his approach, concepts, techniques, and philosophy (Erickson & Rossi 1979; Erickson, 1980g, h, i, & j; Fisch, 1990; Haley, 1973; Lankton & Lankton, 2008/1983, 2007; Lankton, 2004; Rossi, Ryan, & Sharp, 1983; Zeig, 1980; Zeig & Lankton, 1988). I will return to the delineating features of Erickson's approach shortly. First, for the record, I will briefly discuss Milton Erickson, the man.

At the time of his death on Tuesday, March 25, 1980, Erickson was said to have written over 300 professional papers and hypnotized over 30,000 subjects. He was born in Aurum, Nevada, on December 5, 1901. Many readers will probably be familiar with the major accomplishments during his later life: his family of eight children; his many grandchildren; and his worldwide professional impact. For those who are not familiar with his early development and his early professional life, I will provide a brief summary.

It was at age eight that Erickson decided to become a doctor when he grew up, after a family doctor pulled his tooth and gave him a nickel. Around the age of 12 he and some friends learned about hypnosis for the first time from a cheap pamphlet that one of them purchased. Later, he learned techniques of deep introspection that would come to serve him well in his professional life.

He developed infantile paralysis of polio in August 1919, at age 17. He recalled hearing the physicians explain to his mother that her son would not live to see another sunset (personal communication, August, 1974). He indicated that he felt great anger that a mother should be told such a thing about her son. When his family members came into his room after meeting with the doctors, he instructed them to arrange the furniture in a particular way. The rearranged furniture allowed him to see out the west window. Erickson said that he would be "damned if I would die without seeing one more sunset" (personal communication, August, 1974; Rossi, Ryan, & Sharp, 1983, p. 10). Of course, he lived. This experience was powerful in forming Erickson's worldview.

His pre-college years were filled with hours and days of concentration and contemplation. Having survived the predicted death, Erickson was told he would never walk again. He had no sensation or control below his neck. Yet, not being of the mind to accept such speculation without challenge, he spent hours learning to discover feelings and sensations in those muscles not completely destroyed by polio. Erickson learned to revivify and *retrieve experiential* memories of shoveling, hoeing, and so on.

Within a year, he had regained the use of his upper torso and was up on crutches. His later success resulted in having completely regained the use of his legs and his ability to walk and pedal a bicycle around his undergraduate campus. He explained all of these successes to the act of discovering the experiential resources and doing so by appealing to simple, previously learned skills such as using a shovel or a hand hoe. Sufficiently revivifying his use of such tools gradually gave him the access to his motor skills. These episodes of willful intention and the lessons he took from them shaped his professional approach in many ways. He crystallized for himself a path of overcoming one's real or perceived limitations no matter how serious.

In time, Erickson began a premed curriculum at the University of Wisconsin. He actually began officially practicing hypnosis as an undergraduate and was considerably capable by the time he graduated in 1928 with his medical degree. He met and studied hypnosis with Clark Hull who later sponsored him in his internship. As he studied hypnosis in a class taught by Hull, Erickson first began to recognize the difference in the existing view of hypnosis and how it works and what he learned from his own life experience. He did not think, as he was being taught, that the key to hypnosis was suggestion (planted in the unconscious), but rather that the key was developing the experiential resources needed in each particular context.

Erickson interned at Colorado Psychopathic Hospital in child psychiatry and then began working as a senior psychiatrist at Rhode Island State Hospital. In the spring of 1934, he began as the head of psychiatric research at Wayne County General hospital in Eloise, Michigan. Eloise was home to 40,000 psychiatric patients! At that time he began openly practicing and writing about hypnosis. In 1939 he became an associate professor at the Wayne University College of Medicine. He held the position of full professor in Wayne University's Social Service Department and Michigan State College's clinical psychology program.

Dr. Erickson moved to Phoenix in the summer of 1948 in order to find a climate that would reduce his sensitivity to allergens. He worked in the Arizona State Hospital for a period and then went into private practice. Erickson contracted a second type of polio or post-polio syndrome, in 1953. At this time he lost the use of muscles in his back, diaphragm, abdomen, left leg, right arm, mouth, and tongue. In that state, however, he still continued to work with patients and professionals from around the world. Some were ongoing students and some only visited briefly. Among them were such luminaries as Aldous Huxley, Margaret Mead, and Gregory Bateson. Hundreds of well-known psychiatrists, psychologists, and therapists worked with him or visited him including Herbert Speigel, Lawrence Kubie, Seymour Hershman, Irving Secter, Lynn Cooper, Theodore Sarbin, Theodore X. Barber, Andre Weitzenhoffer, Martin Orne, Ernest Hilgard, Jay Haley, Daniel Goleman, Ernest Rossi, Robert Pearson, Sid Rosen, Moshe Feldenkrais, Jeffrey Zeig, myself, and many others.

Erickson once remarked that these physical limitations had also made him more observant. The skills he developed for his own survival he utilized in his observation of others. He became vigilant of the minute muscle movements people employ and found them to be revealing of information that had bearing on clinical issues (Haley, 1967). Erickson said, "My tone deafness has forced me to pay attention to inflections in the voice. This means I'm less distracted by the content of what people say. Many patterns of behavior are reflected in the way a person says something rather than in what he says" (Haley, 1967, p. 2). This keen sense of observation of meaningful patterns of behavior is yet another hallmark that distinguishes Erickson's approach to therapy and hypnosis from most other therapies.

There are several in-depth biographical works on Erickson; this discussion is not intended to summarize or replace them (Haley, 1993; Erickson & Keeney, 2006; Rossie & Ryan, 1985). To explain an Ericksonian approach to therapy and the use of hypnosis and therapy, it is important to establish the absolute necessity of retrieving experiential resources by means of the hypnotic experience. His early recovery from polio, in retrospect, had become the acid test of those concepts. While such a perspective may seem reasonable to many therapists of today, this notion was at odds with traditional psychiatry during much of Erickson's professional life. This approach calls for an active, that is, *strategic*, and participatory therapist—a far cry from an analyst who attempted to be invisible behind a couch.

RATIONALE AND PHILOSOPHY

Erickson's work spanned 50 years and 30,000 clients (Lankton & Lankton, 2008/1983, p. xiii) who came from a broad background: rich, poor; single, married; adults, children; "neurotic," "psychotic"; inpatient, outpatient; urban, rural; and educated, illiterate. Derived from and used with this rich diversity, there are several tenets that affect the practice of therapy as well as the way in which problems and people are viewed.

Assessment and Treatment Planning

"It is not surprising to find at the heart of Erickson's work a diagnostic framework that beats to the rhythm of today's systems and communication theories" (Lankton & Lankton, 2008/1983, p. 28). Erickson formulated and used a relationship and family approach to treating individuals long before it was fashionable. His approach is apparently rooted in the awareness that people operate from internal maps of the world and that these have been learned. These internal guidelines contain rules for interaction, experience, and perception, and these constitute internal experiential resources. In addition, our internal maps will contain learned limitations regarding how we each interact, perceive, and experience the world.

It is perhaps only of minor significance that Dr. Erickson was a pioneer in applying this sort of diagnostic framework. His early writings indicate that he was also well versed in psychodynamic theory. It will be shown later that he occasionally discussed matters such as defense mechanisms and other analytic-dynamic concepts. However, he was reluctant to codify his model of the human mind or human conduct. He would frequently tell students that he made up a new approach for each client. To some degree, this must certainly have been an exaggeration. However, he was sensitive to the unique needs of each individual and did tailor his communication and interventions to that person.

Nevertheless, we can see at a higher level of analysis repeated patterns in his behavior. Before examining these, it is important to mention that Dr. Erickson's work must be considered more than a collection of techniques and patterns. He was a very careful observer, diagnostician, and was a consummate professional who kept careful notes. While it is somewhat easy to understand the interventions that he used, it is more difficult to recognize the diagnostic mindset that he held while using these interventions.

As any trained health care professional should do, Erickson kept detailed case files that recorded his observations, assessments, diagnosis, interventions, and the client's responses to those interventions. He referred to his case files before each session and entered progress notes as soon as possible after each session. While his diagnostic histories were not obtained from a chronology of psychosocial events, they were obtained by careful observation and a selective history of the client's current life context and relationships (personal communication, August, 1975).

Utilization of Client Behavior

Utilization was one of the hallmarks of Erickson's work. Utilization is a process of using the client's energy, point of view, skills, and potentials. "Whatever the patient presents to you in the office, you really ought to use" (Erickson & Rossi, 1981, p. 16). *Utilization* is a term that Erickson used to depict his approach in two important areas. One is the here-and-now use of material presented from the client. If a client demonstrates relaxation, tension, talkativeness, silence, questioning, passivity, movement, stillness, fear, confidence, and so forth, it is to be accepted and used (that is, the client would be directed to continue it) to further the therapeutic movement in a natural way. Tension and "resistance" are not seen as or labeled as such, but rather, are accepted and in some manner used to facilitate a context for change. If a mother, father, and child cling closely to one another, rather than attempting to spatially separate them and calling their resultant hesitation or anxiety "resistance," the therapist may ask them to let the child hold them even closer together with each arm as the interview takes place. This is using the here-and-now behavior to increase the joining and the comfort of the client as well as to reduce the discomfort or anxiety that any other intervention would create.

The second manner in which utilization is intended to be understood applies to using the potential abilities each client brings to the session

(Erickson, 1981, p. 17). Using the latent resources each person brings to a session will allow for a rich diversity in a "typical" therapy session. Each person, for instance, can fantasize, recall, regress, anticipate, relax, forget, imagine, alter consciousness, and so forth, and, using these natural abilities, the client and therapist can cooperate in developing a wide range of helpful contexts for change.

Speak the Client's Own Experiential Language

It follows from the utilization approach that therapists must "speak the client's own experiential language" and "meet them at their model of the world" (Lankton & Lankton, 2008/1983, p. 5). He states, "therefore, you ought to start simply and let the patients elaborate in accord with their own personality needs—not in accord with your concepts of what is useful to them" (Erickson, 1981, p. 12). Communicating in this manner requires that the therapist be flexible in his or her manner. This behavioral flexibility is to be used in the service of matching the client's type of language, conceptual and family orientation, cultural background, and even the client's speed of speaking, bodily posture in movement, and breathing rate, when possible. Dr. Erickson himself had difficulty in moving his limbs, however, first-hand observation of his behavior revealed that he would change other nonverbal behavior to be in rhythm with his clients (Lankton, 2003/1980).

Reduction of Resistance

Several aspects of Erickson's approach can be viewed as components that reduce resistance. These include his attempt to speak the client's language, utilization of the material given rather than confront or block the material given, introduce ambiguity, allow the client's personal interpretation of the ambiguity to temporarily prevail, avoid labels, initially seek very small changes in the therapeutic direction, interpret and reframe client behavior in such a way as to make it appear positive, and so on. By blending therapeutic intervention and guidance with the client's own predisposition for movement, emotion, and thought, Ericksonian therapy can provide very little for clients to resist. A good analogy to help understand this type of interaction with clients is to compare it to the martial arts. Some aspects of conventional therapy might be compared to the confrontation in the martial art of karate, while Ericksonian therapy could be compared to approaches such as in tai chi or aikido (Ueshiba, 1991). In karate, the practitioner learns to block and punch in order to defend against the aggression of the opponent. In tai chi or aikido, the practitioner learns to use the forward movement and energy of the opponent to reduce conflict without aggression. Compare Erickson's view to that of the founder of aikido: "Regarding technique, it is necessary to develop a strategy that utilizes all the physical conditions and elements that are directly at hand. . . . When your opponent wants to pull you must learn to anticipate and direct such a pull" (Ueshiba, 1991, p. 35).

Flexibility and Direct Communication

It's important to note that not all clients bring resistance to therapy. Some clients are highly motivated and cooperative and simply seek the tools they need for change. Other clients commonly seen present a great deal of defensiveness and poor communication or cooperation skills. A hallmark of doing therapy in a fashion that was representative of Erickson's work is the skill of being flexible—that is, the ability to effect change in the most rapid manner despite adapting to the type of client who arrives in the office. When a client arrives who is cooperative, communicates well, and is motivated for change, it is most appropriate to use direct communication, direct hypnotic suggestion, and decisive non-evasive behavior. Dr. Erickson was an expert at this sort of communication. In fact, it can be shown that he used that type of communication for the longest period of his professional career.

The principle of utilization alone dictates that if a *congruent* client comes requesting information and ideas, the therapist ought to take the direct and non-evasive posture that will help fulfill the client's learning needs as soon as possible. For such a client, using indirect, ambiguous, or metaphoric techniques for anything other than illustrating a point with greater clarity would conceivably be an injustice. In this type of direct communication, Erickson was well equipped.

In other words, when initially working with a client who arrives in the office presenting a good deal of motivation, a history of rich personal and interpersonal resources, and is a good communicator, the use of indirect suggestion or metaphor would be less efficient than the use of direct suggestion and non-ambiguous communication. Once again the Ericksonian therapist should be flexible enough to respond by matching these communication signals with similar communication.

Similarly, referring to the principle of utilization, when a client comes to the office who is argumentative, condescending, and competitive, the model provided by Erickson prescribes that therapy should allow the client to win the argument, be one up, and win the competition. An approach of direct communication may provide the best target against which such clients can argue, criticize, and compete. For these clients, the introduction of ambiguity and indirect suggestion could conceivably be inappropriate because it would provide no solid content for the continuance of that client's skill set (regardless of how self-defeating it might be).

However, beyond the context of interview management and after such a client was in trance, then the use of indirect techniques might be most appropriate. This is in part due to the fact that such clients are often not able to easily bring forth the necessary positive experiences to promote change. In these circumstances, indirect techniques become valuable because of the role they play in stimulating thought. To use a colorful analogy, one might say that the mental search that is necessary to personalize and make sense of the ambiguity of indirect techniques is analogous to the active stirring around inside a "junk drawer" to locate a lost object. Rearranging the items of random "junk" often reveals treasures that have been overlooked. In that same way, the listeners of indirect suggestion, binds, anecdote, and metaphor turns over various ideas in their mind in order to discover the best meaning to give the ambiguity. This act of examining and re-examining ideas often yields ideas, methods, and avenues for retrieving desired therapeutic experiences.

Finally, a fourth example would be the case of a client who enters therapy with the customary ambivalence, relatively more impoverished background of resource experiences, moderate communication skills, but encumbered by various learned limitations. Such clients are not particularly compliant nor do they fully understand how to locate and reassociate various experiential resources. Such clients perhaps represent the majority of customary outpatient mental health patients. With these clients a mixture of both direct and indirect suggestion is the most logical way to proceed. Indirect suggestions, anecdotes, binds, and metaphor help listeners create a conditional mental search and tentative understanding. This creates expectancy in the mind of the listener that helps them bring a solid understanding to any subsequent direct communication that follows. This pattern of using indirection followed by direct suggestion, for most clients, will usually prove to be the most efficient both prior to and during trance experiences.

It has been three decades since the death of Dr. Erickson. Yet, some individuals in the therapeutic community may be under the impression that Erickson's most distinctive feature was his use of indirect communication. This would be an incorrect assumption. The most distinctive feature about Erickson's work would likely be best stated in the terms *flexibility* and *utilization*. While other features are also predominately important in his work—such as taking a nonpathological approach, trying to get the client moving as soon as possible, being active and strategic in the therapy, and emphasizing the present and future development of the client rather than the historical past—*flexibility* and *utilization* were the hallmarks of Dr. Erickson's work throughout the course of his career.

Indirection and Ambiguity

Indirection is an orientation to offering ideas that Erickson developed in the last few decades of his career. It became a well-known principle of his approach (Erickson & Rossi, 1980a; Haley, 1963, 1973, 1967; Watzlawick, Weakland, & Fisch, 1974; Fisch, Weakland, & Segal, 1982; Lankton &

Lankton, 2008/1983) in the last half decade before his death. One aspect of indirection is the latitude it provides for each client's own experience and thinking. The use of ambiguity can sometimes instill a certain curiosity that can give rise to a degree of pleasant mental excitement toward change. Rather than detracting from communication, ambiguity often enhances it. This applies not only to hypnosis but also to normal communication conducted with families in waking state conversation.

Perhaps the vast majority of clients that are seen in outpatient psychotherapy are neither highly motivated nor good communicators—nor are they extremely rigid poor communicators. Instead, it might be fair to say that the vast majority of clients for many therapists, especially those in outpatient settings, are only moderately good communicators who are ambivalent about changing and somewhat defensive about their lack of experiential resources. For these individuals, therapy often results in defensiveness and an inability for them to identify and retrieve the needed resources for change. In situations such as these, indirect techniques are often most helpful. Their helpfulness lies in the manner in which they engage the client. They facilitate a mental search process while reducing defensiveness by disguising the desired goal. When clients identify a "fit" between what the suggestion has hinted and their own personal history, the experiential options are expanded. Since they have not had to comply with the therapist's directions, clients who respond to indirection have developed their own answer or their own resource actions from, so to speak, within themselves (Lankton & Lankton, 2008/1983).

It is important that the reader bear in mind that indirection does not constitute a defining feature of Erickson's approach. It constitutes one of the pillars that he relied upon in his career, having perfected it in his later years. However, there is a danger in promoting the use of indirect techniques among inexperienced therapists or professionals using hypnosis. The danger is found not in the technique itself, but rather in an attitude that is occasionally inferred by would-be practitioners who have not thoroughly learned the clinical logic behind indirect techniques. Using indirect techniques correctly and effectively takes a great deal of work and study. It is unfortunately too common that I hear students of an indirect approach state that a therapist only needs to simply "trust their unconscious" and tell clients content that is spontaneously delivered.

The model displayed by Erickson was anything but a "fly-by-the-seat-of-your-pants" or spontaneous approach. Erickson worked out the wording of his inductions and his early stories over a period of dozens of drafts. He would write out, for example, a 20-page induction and edit it down to 12 pages. Then he would edit his 12-page induction down to 7 pages. Eventually he would continue the edit until what remained was a page and a half of a well-crafted induction (Haley, 1967). While he was a keen observer, he did not interpret meaning to his observations flippantly. He was a strong critic of people who claim to be mind readers (personal communication, August, 1978). He developed his understanding and observational skills over the period of many years and built those understandings on a foundation that originated from a deeply personal insight into his own motor behavior. Therapists who believe they can replicate that sort of observational talent are likely to be grossly mistaken.

Being aware that one will not be as perceptive as Erickson means that those professionals who wish to apply his work in their therapy will need to augment their face-to-face communication with clients. There will be a need for more verbal confirmation from clients. And too, there may be a need for the use of other assessment tools. Even simple tools like the Interpersonal Check List (Leary, 1957) can provide valuable insight about the range of behavior a client is capable of producing for those of us who are not as perceptive as Erickson.

The use of tools of indirection includes metaphor, indirect suggestion, therapeutic binds, anecdote, and ambiguous function assignments (Lankton & Lankton, 2008/1983, 1986). In contrast to direct techniques and direct suggestion, indirect techniques are difficult to learn, understand, and use. Therefore, I have often written about and taught these techniques in my professional publications and workshops. It is my intention to provide a sufficient articulation of these ambiguous techniques so as to make possible to construct well-conceived empirical research studies about them and to help therapists use them wisely. Lacking such careful articulation, these techniques will simply be lost to history. Therefore, I will provide further details and an illustration about these lesser understood and practiced techniques of Erickson's work.

Hypnotic Language

Hypnotic language refers to verbal and nonverbal communication that elicits unconscious responses in a single listener or in multiple listeners. Traditionally, when one speaks of hypnotic language, it means direct suggestion, and means that the hypnotist makes a clear and direct request for a certain response. For example, "Close your eyes. Listen to everything I say. Follow my suggestions completely." In addition, however, when one speaks of hypnotic language, it may mean a form of indirect suggestion where the relationship between the operator's suggestion and the subject's response is less obvious. Indirect language can also include forms of confusion, anecdote, and metaphor. For example, "Your conscious mind may not immediately realize how much your unconscious mind will learn. You might enjoy how much you learn sooner or later."

Direct suggestion can be defined as the language that elicits an unconscious response to a stated goal. Direct suggestion gets best results when the operator's prestige and authority is high and the principles of repetition, along with the evocation of ideosensory and ideomotor processes are used (Weitzenhoffer, 1957). Sometimes these are enhanced by goal-directed fantasy that is often recognized as the basis of direct suggestion (Barber, Spanos, & Chaves, 1974).

Erickson states that "much of hypnotic psychotherapy can be accomplished indirectly" (Erickson & Rossi, 1981, p. 13). Indirect suggestion is hypnotic language that is recognized for being ambiguous, vague, and more permissive in nature. Responses to indirect suggestion are recognized as being a function of the subject's personal need, and, perhaps because of this, they may be more effective, or at least experienced as being more relevant, than direct suggestion at an individual level. The rationale for using indirect suggestion is also characterized by a number of basic features that are of particular interest:

- Indirect suggestion permits the subject's individuality, previous experience, and unique potentials to become manifest;
- The classical psychodynamics of learning with processes like association, contiguity, similarity, contrast checking, and so forth, are all involved on a unconscious level;
- Indirect suggestion tends to bypass conscious criticism and learned limitations. Because of this it can be more effective and long lasting than direct suggestion.

Indirect suggestion may be successfully used with subjects who are awake; in waking state its suggestive influence is much greater than that of a direct suggestion. It frequently exerts an effective influence on people who do not yield to direct suggestion, as was pointed out by V. Bekhterev and colleagues (Bekhterev, 1998). It could be said that the stronger suggestion is the one that is more concealed.

Language can be direct, indirect, confusing, anecdotal, logical, rational, poetic, and metaphoric. Let me say that again, all language is hypnotic language and it varies by degree of effectiveness. If we classify communication by degrees of effective hypnotic response that it produces, we would be able to place all communication into a continuum of hypnotic language—from minimally effective to powerfully effective. We can measure this effectiveness in several ways by answering some simple questions of both low and highly hypnotizable subjects: How soon does the person respond to the language? How long does the effect last? How resistant to change is the response? How much energy, effort, or repetition must be used to obtain the response?

In any event, the goal in using hypnotic language is to elicit experience in the listener. The goal is not, as some uninformed people might think, to place an idea in the subconscious. Again, the goal of language is to elicit experience: cognitive, perceptual, emotional, and behavioral experience.

Depathologizing

Since problems are not thought to be "inside" a person's head, there is a depathologizing of people (Fisch, 1990). Problems are thought to be the result of trying to move toward a more normal state in an unfolding life cycle (Haley, 1973, p. 150). Ericksonian therapy attempts to avoid labels and redefine any possible stigma attached to a client's presenting problem. In a dramatic example of this, Erickson once had a young withdrawn woman with a previously embarrassing gap in her teeth. He encouraged her to learn to propel water through that gap. He eventually convinced her to shoot water at a young man who had shown some interest in her and whom she had avoided. The results of this interaction eventually led to the courtship between these two young people (Haley, 1973). By allowing this girl to continue to avoid contact with others, and by redefining the gap in her teeth as something enjoyable rather than a deformity, he was able to avoid the obvious resistances that could have been created by an approach to therapy that wished to teach her to become assertive and proud "despite her problem." Ironically, she did become assertive and proud but was able to do so without having to first consider her problems as a negative liability she was going to have to overcome in the course of therapy (Haley, 1973).

Therapy is directed toward helping clients contribute to a creative rearrangement in their relationships so that developmental growth is maximized. Accompanying the reduction of the pathology oriented assessment is a corresponding reduction in so-called resistance.

Creating a Context for Change

Additionally, in Ericksonian therapy, the therapist is active and shares responsibility for initiating therapeutic movement and "creating a context in which change can take place" (Dammann, 1982). This is often facilitated by introducing material into the therapy session and by the use of suggestion, metaphor, and even extramural assignments. That is, a therapist may not wait until clients spontaneously bring up material but rather may invite or challenge clients to grow and change by creating a context in which it can occur. It would probably be most accurate to say that an Ericksonian therapist does not consider himself or herself an expert on the client who appears in the office, but rather tries to be an expert for creating a context for that client to change. That context can be didactic outpatient psychotherapy, psychotherapy done in hypnosis, family therapy, couples therapy, homework assignments, or combinations of all of the above. But it is working with the unique client to develop a context that works for them that constitutes another aspect of the flexibility that is a hallmark of Ericksonian therapy.

Getting the Client Moving as Soon as Possible

Ericksonian therapy is interested in getting clients active and moving (Zeig, 1980). This movement can begin with very small incremental changes inside the office and later be magnified into greater behavioral changes in their lives outside the office. Hypnotherapy and the use of direct suggestion, anecdotes, therapeutic metaphors, and indirect suggestions are ways of conversing with clients to help create the impetus during sessions to carry out new relational behaviors or congruently engage in the homework assignments. It's conceivable, for example, that a client would be taught during a session to begin moving a finger when he hears his wife speak. This simple behavior could then be leveraged to having him turn his head to make eye contact with his wife when she speaks outside the session.

Assignments are often given in order to have clients carry out agreed-upon behaviors between the sessions. It is from the learning brought by new actions and not from insight or understanding that change develops. It may be, in fact, that "change leads to insight" (Dammann, 1982, p. 195). Consequently, clients' understanding or insight about a problem is not of central importance. The matters of central importance are the clients' participation in new experiences and transactions in which they congeal developmentally appropriate relational patterns.

Present and Future Orientation

Ericksonian therapy is future oriented and is centered upon an integration of family therapy and individual hypnotherapy, though these areas are often seen as extremes with very little convergence. The influence of Erickson's approach grew in these two areas independently as it provided examples for the philosophical work of Bateson and other epistemological thinkers who emphasized the need to depart from a model of linear causality associated with the medical model of therapy (Fisch, 1990).

The Ericksonian-strategic approach is a method of working with clients emphasizing common, even unconscious, natural abilities and talents. This is in distinct contrast to conventional psychotherapy approaches that place an emphasis upon dysfunctional aspects of clients an attempt to analyze, interpret, or develop insight for them during therapy sessions. Instead, it works to frame change in ways that reduce resistance, reduce dependence upon therapy, bypass the need for insight, and expand creative adjustment to developmental demands, while removing the presenting problem and allowing individuals to take full credit for changes achieved in therapy.

In the development of most approaches to psychotherapy, there has been considerable effort to elaborate a theory that will guide clinical procedure. While practice needs to be informed by theory and research, the clinical interventions developed from theory or research often are restrictive in the range of behaviors prescribed for the therapist. This appears particularly true for psychoanalytically oriented therapies that until very recently have continued to hold a position of dominance in the medical and psychological communities.

Erickson and Rossi (2008) identified the limitations of these therapies as arising from three general assumptions:

- Therapy based on observable behavior and related to the present and future circumstances of the client is often viewed as superficial and lacking depth when compared to therapies that seek to restructure clients' understandings of the distant past.
- The same approach to therapy (e.g., classical analysis, gestalt, Transactional Analysis, or non-directive therapy) is not appropriate for all clients in all circumstances.
- Effective therapy occurs through an interpretation and explanation of a client's inner life based on the assumptions of the given theory. Change, from this perspective, occurs mainly through insight by a client into his or her behavior.

These assumptions deny the context of the problem, the unique learnings, experiences, and resources of clients, and the type of symptom presented. Most therapies require, if only inadvertently, that clients adapt to the therapist's worldview when it may not be in their best interests to do so. From early in his life, Erickson began to challenge traditional notions, expectations, and limitations placed on him.

We can see examples of this difference even in the initial contact that Erickson has with clients. Erickson felt that focusing on childhood psychosocial history, to the exclusion of the client's daily life, contradicts basic experience. Events in daily life can have a profound influence in the development of character or personality. As Erickson & Rossi (2008) correctly point out, these events do not need to be considered extensions of earlier unresolved infantile traumas in order to be understood.

While people have memories, perceptions, feelings, and so forth regarding their past, current realities impinge on them that affect their daily and future interactions in the world. Preoccupation with the past and a disregard of present and future needs unnecessarily prolong and complicate the process of therapy. In fact, the phenomenon of selective recall may provide the client with a great deal of apparent facts about the past that parallel the present problem. While Erickson himself never said so, one might go so far as to speculate whether or not memories of the past constitute a sort of metaphor for the client's present experiences.

In any event, a hallmark of an Ericksonian approach is an emphasis on current interpersonal relationships and their influence on the development and resolution of problems. While an individual may have developed a symptomatic behavior in the distant past, the Ericksonian view focuses on how the problem is maintained in the present. Thus, in this approach, the unique interpersonal interactions in the client's present life are of primary importance, rather than a reliance on the application of a rigid theory and technique.

CHANGES IN TREATMENT APPROACH OVER TIME

When considering this emphasis on interpersonal focus, it's important to note the difference between Erickson's early career practices and his later career developments. The field of psychotherapy in hypnosis has witnessed controversy about Erickson's approach. Some individuals would claim that Erickson's later students misunderstood his approach (Hammond, 1988). Because some individuals emphasized techniques of indirection and ignored Erickson's use of techniques that were more direct, a schism developed. It was clear to individuals who studied directly with Erickson, rather than those who simply learned about him through his writings, that the schism did not need to exist.

Individuals who studied with Erickson early in his career witnessed a man who was highly influenced by the prevailing psychoanalytic theory and the style of authoritarian-directed hypnosis that existed. At that point in his career, Erickson used a great deal of repetition, redundancy, and direct suggestion. Later in his career, Erickson evolved from this authoritarian approach and changed to a more ambitious style of therapy. The more permissive and ambiguous approach to hypnosis and psychotherapy that Erickson demonstrated in his later years was not the result of Erickson mentally and physically deteriorating, as some have intimated (Hammond, 1984). Erickson specifically addresses the issue of his change and the rationale for his change in his writings. He had a well-thought out and logical reason for including more forms of interaction and permissiveness in his psychotherapy and hypnosis. He felt that it was important to good therapy to allow clients a greater latitude of understanding. He believed that indirect techniques facilitated the client developing their own experience rather than complying to the demands of the therapist (Erickson and Rossi, 1980c).

Perhaps the professional who studied with Erickson for the longest period of continuous time was Jay Haley. Haley was witness to Erickson's earlier approach to change as well as his later approach to change. This distinguishes him from those who experienced Erickson either in the earlier or in the later decades of his career. Haley did not consider Erickson's later emphasis upon indirection in hypnosis and therapy a result of his physical deterioration (incidentally, there was certainly no evidence of mental deterioration in Erickson). If he did, in fact, develop the indirect approach because he was physically ailing in his later years, readers might take a lighthearted humor in the recognition that a reliance upon indirect techniques may very well reduce stress on the therapist but it appears to increase the therapist's effectiveness with many clients! What could be better? In any case, we can see the articulation of this evolution, from a reliance upon direct communication to a more indirect approach to therapy and an evolution from a strongly authoritarian to a more permissive interpersonal posture in Erickson's own words if we study the entire body of his written work.

CHANGES IN TREATMENT DURATION

In the early 1950s, we see several cases during which Erickson took months and years. The case of the man with a "fat lip" took upwards of 11 months (Erickson and Rossi, 1979, p. 224) and the case of the "February Man" from Michigan took far longer—up to two years (Erickson, 1980a, pp. 525–542). While it is true that Erickson made himself available to clients for an indefinite period of time while he lived in Phoenix, his published cases became shorter in duration. In 1973 we find the case of the eight-year-old "stomper" that took two hours (Haley, 1973, p. 219). Various cases of his "shock" technique in 1973 entailed one- to two-hour long sessions (Erickson & Rossi, 1980a, p. 447). In general, the movement to brief therapy progressed continually and became prominent in his practice in the late 1960s and beyond.

Changes in Erickson's Conceptualization of Symptoms

Let's consider some changes in the view of symptoms from a psychoanalytic view to an interactional view. From his earliest years as a psychiatrist at least until 1954, Erickson took a traditional analytic view of neurosis and various symptoms. He said the development of neurotic symptoms "constitutes behavior of a defensive, protective character" (Erickson, 1980c, p. 149). At this early point in his career, he had not fully developed a theory that was opposed to the prevailing traditional understanding of behavior.

By the mid-1960s, his view had become much more interactional. Perhaps this was a result of his collaboration with Jay Haley, Gregory Bateson, John Weakland, and the Palo Alto Communication Project. In any case, Erickson writes, in 1966, "Mental disease is the breaking down of communication between people" (Erickson, 1980d, p. 75). However, by the end of his career, he had moved even further from the analytic and the communications or systems theory of disease. He states, "Symptoms are forms of communication" and "cues of developmental problems that are in the process of becoming conscious" (Erickson & Rossi, 1979, p. 143). His evolution of thought about problems became less and less focused on them as pathological artifacts until, in the end, symptoms could be seen as communication signals of desired directions of growth. Erickson even went so far as to take such signals to be a request for change, albeit unconscious contracts for therapeutic engagement. However, in today's world, Erickson would have been restricted by requirements and considerations of informed consent, of course.

Cure Accomplished by Reassociation of Experience

A focus on the psychosocial past can often reveal moments of learned limitation. For example, a historical event may reveal the most intense example of a time when a patient learned to avoid expressing a certain emotion that is still lacking in the present. Exploring the past events and traumas can be the basis for some types of psychotherapy, but that should not be therapy's exclusive focus. Ericksonian therapy is based on identifying client strengths and increasing the possibility of new learnings and experiences that can be used for solving problems in the client's present life. The retrieval or building of that missing emotional experience would be central in the Ericksonian approach. In addition, his approach focuses on orienting clients to solutions necessary for future developmental changes.

At least one area in which Erickson never wavered in the course of his career was his view of what constituted "cure." I suspect this was a result of his personal experience overcoming paralysis. He learned as a young adult that experiential resources created change. As early as 1948 Erickson recognized that cure was not the result of suggestion but rather resulted from the reassociation of experiences (Erickson, 1980e, p. 38). In the later years of his career, we find this theme repeated again and again (Erickson & Rossi, 1979; Erickson & Rossi, 1980b, p. 464; Erickson & Rossi, 1981).

Changes in Use of Hypnotic Suggestion

As mentioned, professionals who studied with Erickson early in his career purport a different orientation to therapy than those who studied with him during his later years. In a 1957 transcript of induction, we find Erickson's redundant use of words like *sleep* as in the following quote, "Now I want you to go deeper and deeper asleep" (Haley, 1967, p. 54). In addition, his authoritative approach can be found in this same transcript represented with the statement, "*I can put* you in any level of trance" [italics mine] (Haley, 1967, p. 64). However, by 1976 Erickson believed indirection to be a "significant factor" (Erickson, Rossi, & Rossi, 1976, p. 452) in his work. Furthermore, by 1981 Erickson clearly states that he "offers" ideas and suggestions (Erickson & Rossi, 1981, pp. 1–2) and explicitly adds, "I don't like this matter of telling a patient I want you to get tired and sleepy" (Erickson & Rossi 1981, p. 4). With regard to his use of indirection, this appears to be clear evidence that it evolved to occupy a prominent place in his practice to a point in the late 1970s when Erickson had all but abandoned his earlier techniques of redundancy and authoritarianism during induction.

BASICS INTERVENTIONS OF THE APPROACH

It is difficult to categorize Erickson's customary approach to therapy—that is, the approach that he most commonly used. There are a wide range of case examples where the technique used was never repeated. On the other hand, there are some interventions that were clearly used repeatedly such as the February Man story and commands delivered within that story. Others include the use of reframing, the use of indirect suggestion to induce trance and retrieve experiences, the use of confusion technique, structured amnesia, and the use of rehearsals done through visual imagination and trance.

Speaking the Client's Language and Matching Behavior

Erickson's own explanations were often frustrating to many of his students, as he insisted upon sharing wisdom in a rather folksy manner. For instance, asked what the most important thing was in therapy, he would comment, "Speak the client's own experiential language." When asked for the next most important thing to do, he commented, "Put one foot in the client's world and leave one foot in your own" (personal communication, August, 1975). Such comments seemed to side step conventional scientific language and left one wondering if he would eventually come to add more. He never would.

The topic of matching the behavior of the client is a logical extension of speaking the client's language. Certainly speaking clients' language is matching their verbal behavior and way of expressing themselves. There has also been a good bit of discussion in the last three decades about matching the client's physical behavior. It is not accurate however to say that Erickson would find it appropriate in his practice to mirror the behavior of all of the clients he saw. There are many examples of cases that have been published about Erickson's work in which he clearly took an interpersonal posture that was dissimilar than that of his clients (Haley, 1973). For example, there is a case of a woman who had very low self-esteem and was overweight—in this case, Erickson initially took a role that would be described as hostile and dominant. In another case, a man who was a flute player saw Erickson because of his enlarged and swollen lower lip. This client was extremely hostile and critical of Erickson—in this case, Erickson took a role that would be described as submissive and self-critical. In other cases he played a role that could be described as bossy and told parents they were to allow him to make all of the decisions about their son. In still another case, Erickson played a very critical role when he turned and stomped on the feet of a young girl who felt obsessed about the size of her growing feet. Each of these cases and more can be found in the *Uncommon Therapy* casebook (Haley, 1973).

So what are we to make of the allegation that Erickson matched the behavior of his clients in a symmetrical fashion when so many cases illustrate that he did not? The answer is quite simple. Once again, the key is that Erickson demonstrated flexibility in his approach. However, there are guidelines for matching that may not be quite so evident at first glance. In each of the cases I cited before, Erickson took a complementary role rather than a symmetrical role in his interpersonal posture with these clients. I'd like to illustrate this with the following explanation. Assume a simple bell curve that describes the range of client behavior from, on the left side, extremely flexible or loose behavior through relatively normal behavior in the middle and all the way to extremely rigid behavior on the far right side of the curve. That is to say, behavior that tends to match the cultural norm is in the middle of the bell curve. Each standard deviation to the left-hand side describes increasingly more chaotic behavior that would include, for example, moderate to high anxiety, histrionic behavior, hysterical behavior, borderline behavior, and eventually psychotic behavior. Each standard deviation to the right-hand side from the norm would contain examples of increasingly rigid behavior such as, depression, obsession, compulsion, narcissism, and paranoia, until finally one reached a paranoid personality type behavior. I am not concerned about the exact ordering of these diagnostic labels. Rather, I am concerned with the notion that behavior can be extremely chaotic or extremely rigid and that we could look at this on a continuum in which we find culturally normative behavior located in the middle of the bell curve.

Once we have constructed this mental map, we have a good way to better understand the logic of using the concept of matching in Ericksonian approaches to therapy and hypnosis. Using Erickson's successful behavior with clients as a model, the following conclusion could be drawn. Those clients that fall, loosely, within a standard deviation both sides of normative behavior would be met with a *symmetrical* matching. That is, the body posture of the therapist would match the body posture of the client. This behavioral matching could be done with extreme attention to detail so the therapist matches the client's movement of limbs, legs, breathing, eye movements, and so forth.

However, once the presentation of the client's behavior exceeds a certain limit beyond the normative and, by comparison, is overly rigid or overly chaotic, the therapist may be well advised to use *complementary* matching instead of symmetrical. For example, if an extremely hostile and rigid prosecuting attorney seeks therapy, matching the client's behavior in a symmetrical fashion may be ill advised. It's extremely possible or likely that such an interpersonal posture would result in a symmetrical escalation of hostilities. Instead, taking a complementary matching position would probably make for a better joining maneuver. The flexibility to allow oneself to initially be in a position of receiving criticism from such a client could be seen as an implementation of the utilization principle.

The conclusion that should be drawn from this discussion is that the initial joining behavior frequently referred to as "matching" has to be considered as a subset to the utilization principle of Ericksonian therapy. There are instances of matching that will establish a symmetrical relationship and cases of matching that will establish a complementary relationship. Finally, the therapeutic indicators that help determine which type of matching will provide the best initial therapeutic union have to do with the degree of rigidity or chaotic behavior exhibited by the client. In addition, the experience of the therapist in dealing with individuals who exhibit a broad range of behavior, and the unique characteristic of any particular client, are the final determinants of when the selection of complementary versus symmetrical matching should take place.

Hypnosis

Hypnosis was part of Erickson's therapy at least as early as 1934 (Haley, 1967, p. 2) and he is probably most recognized as a pioneer and proponent of clinical hypnosis. Erickson stated that hypnosis was "primarily a state in which there is an increased responsiveness to ideas of all sorts" (Erickson & Rossi, 1981, p. 4). However, it should be noted that not all of the Ericksonian therapy models that developed from Erickson's influence have included or emphasized hypnosis. Some practitioners of an Ericksonian approach to therapy (or who borrowed heavily from Erickson's work) emphasize strategic assignments, therapeutic ordeals, or family therapy using paradoxical directives, behavior rehearsal, structured interactions, and direct suggestion, to the exclusion of hypnotherapy and hypnotic indirection (Haley, 1984, 1985a, 1985b, & 1985c; de Shazer, 1985; Lankton, S., 2001).

It is certainly possible to simply have therapeutic "conversations" that do not at first glance resemble formal trance (Matthews, 1985b). However, hypnosis is a useful tool to accomplish certain interview management, continue diagnostic assessment, and stimulate novel thinking, feeling, and resource retrieval within the session. There are a variety of opportunities to introduce hypnosis in Ericksonian therapy and one of these is simply to notice and encourage naturally occurring altered states of consciousness that clients will automatically experience. Whether or not to formally label the experience "trance" is sometimes a debatable issue. Indeed, one of Erickson's primary contributions was an emphasis on the naturally occurring elements of "common everyday trance" and demystification about trance being an unusual or vulnerable state of consciousness (Erickson &

Rossi, 1976, 1979, 1980b). It "always utilizes such naturalistic modes of functioning; it never imposes anything alien on the patient" (Erickson & Rossi, 1981, p. 5). His work blurred the boundaries between formal trance and "waking" state (Erickson, 1980f). "I am not very greatly concerned about the depth of the trance the patient is in . . ." (Erickson & Rossi, 1981, p. 3). Experiences of searching for meaning in response to an ambiguous or cryptic suggestion can lead to "therapeutic receptivity"—that condition in which clients can discover relevant experiences and facilitate the "answers" for which they are searching (Lankton & Lankton, 2008/1983).

While hypnosis is listed here as an intervention or technique, it is more accurate to think of hypnosis as a *modality for exchanging ideas and stimulating thinking with a client* and concentration on their own experience. "The essential point is that they pay attention, not necessarily to me, but to their own thoughts—especially the thoughts that flash through their mind" (Erickson, 1981, p. 5). As a modality or context for communication, less emphasis is placed on hypnosis itself and instead attention is focused on that which is relevant. Too often, people think of hypnosis as something that the expert practitioner will do *to* them and that it will, in and of itself, cure them or simply remove the troublesome symptom. This is a view of hypnosis Ericksonian practitioners work to dispel in favor of asking clients what resource experiences they need to retrieve while relying upon hypnosis as an aid.

Using Hypnosis with Families

It has been mentioned that not all practitioners of an Ericksonian approach use hypnosis. However, it should be noted that many of the family therapists who embrace an Ericksonian approach to therapy also use hypnosis in their family therapy (Ritterman, 1983; Parsons-Fein, 2004). While that is not the major emphasis of this writing, I offer the following guidelines that have been observed and developed for introducing and using hypnosis in a family session (Lankton & Lankton, 2007/1986).

- Try to initially avoid using hypnosis with the identified patient in a family. This is because family therapists do not wish to reinforce the possible myth that this family member "contains" the problem in the family.
- Protect the identified patient from further exposure to discrimination. Since hypnosis is largely misunderstood by the general public, it is important to be certain that he or she is not seen as "so sick as to require a formidable intervention like hypnosis."
- Avoid playing the role that a rigid family might be assigning—for example, "fix the problem in the 'sick' member."
- Do, however, introduce hypnosis for the purpose of facilitating relief to the person currently experiencing or communicating the most pain.

- If the identified patient also happens to be the client member who is in the most pain, make an exception to the first guideline by offering hypnosis to both the identified patient and the most "healthy" family member or members.

- Hypnosis with two or more individuals at the same time provides a context for building rapport between them (this is especially useful if they are struggling and failing to build a relationship for various reasons).

- Hypnotize all adults in the family. This can be done for the purpose of a stated shared goal or, alternatively, for individual goals that are unique to each individual. This latter type of approach requires greater effort, concentration, and training on the part of the therapists.

Induction of Hypnosis

With regard to introducing trance, it is possible to simply notice the naturally occurring inwardly focused attention of a client and suggest that this experience be intensified. This is not very much different from the often routine suggestion to someone experiencing a particular emotion to "go with that feeling." Though that therapeutic directive is not usually associated with the development of hypnotic trance, per se, formal hypnotic induction need not consist of a break in the normal flow of communication.

This type of conversational induction is usually not considered to be an unusual disruption in the therapeutic process. It often includes additional suggestions for "focusing inward" and deepening absorption. Suggestions such as, "you can close your eyes as you allow yourself to go deeper with that feeling and that experience and perhaps notice that things outside you can seem irrelevant for the moment" and so on. However, the word *trance* or *hypnosis* need not be used at all. Conversational induction underscores the idea that hypnosis is simply a modality for exchanging ideas as are other more familiar interventions.

Therapists use different methods of introducing hypnosis, but the two most common approaches are methods of naturalistic induction (often accompanying an internal fixation) and methods of formal induction (often accompanying an external fixation). The naturalistic induction method involves an elicitation of the unconscious material that accompanies the conscious contract developed and shared with the therapist and usually related to the client's initial request for treatment. Often clients are prepared to become absorbed in a contemplation of their possible gains from therapeutic work. When that occurs, therapists can ask the subject to close their eyes and experience some aspect of this internal resource. That is, the client might mention that he or she would like to overcome depression and feel as lighthearted as he or she once did. When the therapist recognizes the slightest indicator that the client has a memory of feeling lighthearted, it is an opportunity to ask the client to close their eyes and began to recover both the memory and experience of feeling lighthearted. With this very slight alteration of consciousness, hypnosis can be initiated and developed from that conversational beginning. In this case, the induction and subsequent hypnosis represents the immediate therapeutic attempt to perform a naturalistic induction.

As clients increase their internal concentration, they will of course respond in ways that signal their degree of success. In addition to head nodding and head shaking (and the meaning attributed to each), search phenomena are of a broader category. Behaviors in this category range from slight to extreme changes in various reflexes, muscle tone, and skin color. Easily recognized search phenomena indicators include slowed swallow, blink, and breathing reflex, increased skin pallor, and increased muscle lassitude in the cheeks and forehead. This behavior is taken to indicate that clients are experiencing some degree of a sense of fitness between the suggestions and their own personal frame of reference (Lankton & Lankton, 2008/1983, 2007/1986). However, it further demonstrates that clients are not altogether certain that the resources they need are available. Hence, they are searching for further connections between the goals they value and the tools they know they have. In other words, the search phenomena indicate the client's willingness and perceived need to move in the implied direction at the present time.

The nonverbal dialogue with therapists at this subtle level constitutes a sort of unconscious contract development. Again, it occurs by means of ideomotor response to ideas conveyed by therapists who imply successful developmental gains. Clients can also be asked to answer verbally, of course. In so doing, they will often indicate a further elaboration of the presenting conscious contract. This form of gentle induction of hypnosis illustrates that hypnosis is a natural response to communication and problem solving. It tends to demystify hypnosis and promote the notion that it has a rightful place in the realm of natural and ordinary interventions from which therapists can choose. Once again, trance maintenance suggestions and suggestions of deepening are often necessary to facilitate greater internal absorption and the appearance of phenomena usually associated with various trance depths. Although naturalist and conversational inductions often require more skill from the therapist, they require less compliance from the client.

The procedure for a formal induction with external fixation is similar to that used in a traditional ritualistic induction. The subjects are asked to set their attention on some close external object so they might become more absorbed in the process of concentration. As they do, the therapist proceeds with any one of a variety of instructions most suited for the particular client before them: conscious-unconscious dissociation induction, systematic relaxation and deepening, naturalistic, traditional, guided imagery, and so forth. While traditional ritualistic inductions are often contrasted to the conversational or naturalistic induction, it should be noted the selection of suggestions formed with permissive language, indirect suggestions, and therapeutic binds make this sort of formalized inductions distinctly different than those created with direct suggestions. The times-structuring of a formal trance induction separates the trance from what followed and that demarcation can serve to provide security and familiarity to those clients who come to therapy with more rigid expectations of what hypnosis ought to be like.

Often, a formal induction of hypnosis proceeds by asking clients to be seated with their arms and legs uncrossed and their attention focused to a progressive relaxation throughout the body. As the relaxation is deepened, the therapist may even use counting to help the client develop an expectation that their internal focus is also going deeper. This sort of formal induction is perfectly acceptable; however, the aforementioned methods of conversational and naturalistic inductions may be much more consistent with an approach that utilizes the client's immediate presentations and concerns.

In a permissive approach, clients should be offered suggestions with an understanding that they can follow those that are relevant, modify those that can be modified to become relevant, and ignore those suggestions that seem to be irrelevant. All clients, through this type of participation, are responding to their own meaning that they place on the words from the therapist, or in a way, hypnotizing themselves. They are in control of engaging or disengaging from the therapist's influence as a result. It stands to reason, then, that clients will stay in trance as long as the material provided is relevant or appears relevant to their growth concerns.

Formal Induction Sequence Outline

1. *Orient the client to trance.*
   This step involves making certain that the clients are physically, cognitively, and psychologically prepared for the trance.
2. *Fixate attention and rapport.*
   Most frequently clients' attention is fixated on a visual object, story, or body sensation such as relaxation.
3. *Establish a conscious–unconscious dissociation* (Lankton & Lankton, 2008/ 1983, 2007/1986).
   Therapists use conscious-unconscious dissociation language (Lankton & Lankton, 2008/1983, p. 141), including the possible use of anecdote and education about unconscious processes to assist clients in the development of dissociated and polarized attention.

4. *Ratify and deepen the trance.*

   Ratification of the client's process of unconscious search is easily accomplished by helping focus client awareness on the many alterations that occur in their face muscles, reflexes, respiration, and skin coloration. Deepening may be facilitated by several means including confusion, offering small incremental steps, or indirect suggestions, therapeutic binds, and controlled ambiguity.

5. *Utilize trance to elicit experiences and subsequently associate experiences.*

   Therapeutic use of trance includes using those unconscious processes stimulated by induction. The experiences needed are determined by the diagnostic assessment and contracted therapy goals. Experience may be facilitated by the use of indirect suggestion and anecdotes, therapeutic binds, metaphor, guided imagery, direct suggestion, and so forth. Finally, therapists help clients arrange elicited experiences into a network of associations that will help them form a perceptually and behaviorally based map of conduct.

6. *Reorient the client to waking state.*

   Reorientation may be rapid or gradual. At this stage, the therapist has a final opportunity to assist clients in developing amnesia, posthypnotic behavior, and/or other trance phenomena that are part of the treatment plan.

Therapists trained in the Ericksonian approaches are most likely to use a conscious-unconscious dissociation or a conversational induction (Erickson & Rossi, 1979). Such an induction produces the groundwork for further elaboration with ambiguity of indirect suggestion, therapeutic binds, and therapeutic metaphor. A degree of increased dissociation begins to occur in response to comments about unconscious experience. Language such as the following may be used to facilitate that dissociation with the client: "Your conscious mind can listen to the things that I say while your unconscious begins to identify those ideas that are relevant for you." "Your conscious mind may be listening and sorting through your experiences while your unconscious relates in a global fashion to the experiences that you need." And, "your conscious mind may be following a certain train of thought while your unconscious reacts symbolically or follows an entirely different train of thought that's useful for you."

In this manner, therapists direct the conscious mind to experiences that are easily validated and basically true for the client at that time. Thus, the induction is individualized and relevant. Comments regarding the unconscious mind of a client are generally more global, contain a great deal more ambiguity, and will involve an amount of vagueness. This sort of vagueness can easily be elaborated and controlled by the use of therapeutic stories or indirect suggestion.

Hypnotherapeutic interventions strictly aimed toward the verbally shared contract will be understood as relevant by most clients. A clear contract reduces clients' surprise or possible sense of having been deceived. With many clients, this is of concern and ought to be given serious attention. While, with other clients, this is less of a concern due to their understanding that they are seeking the therapist's professional skill, regardless of the specific form it takes.

No matter which of the chosen method of induction, what happens before and after the trance also needs to be considered carefully. After the trance experience is terminated, it may be useful to once again ask clients to engage in the problem-solving communications that had preceded the trance. In this way, resources retrieved during the trance will be further associated to immediately relevant concerns and increase the likelihood that the course of problem solving will be enhanced. Additionally, the entire trance experience is logically embedded in the middle of a structured interaction that is designed to bolster changing individual personality structure and transactional patterns.

The Use of Metaphor as Indirect Intervention

In 1944, Erickson reluctantly published "The Method Employed to Formulate a Complex Story for the Induction of the Experimental Neurosis" (Erickson, 1980b, p. 336). His understanding at that point was that a complex story that paralleled a client's problem could actually heighten the client's discomfort and bring the neurosis closer to the surface. Within a decade, in 1954, he was using "fabricated case histories" of fleeting symptomatology (Erickson, 1980c, p. 152) indicating that at least some of the stories he told had been *confabulated*. Still, almost two decades later in 1973, we see that Erickson provides several examples of case stories for making a therapeutic point (Haley, 1963) and by 1979 he actually used the heading of "metaphor" as a class of interventions (Erickson & Rossi, 1979, p. 49). Again, this movement corresponds to his movement from direct and authoritarian therapy to indirect and permissive therapy.

Uses of Metaphoric Stories

A therapeutic metaphor is *a story with dramatic devices that captures attention and provides an altered framework through which clients can entertain novel experience* (Lankton, 2003/1980; Lankton & Lankton, 2008/1983, 1989, 2007). Metaphor is a form of two-level communication that uses words with multiple connotations and associations so that a client's conscious mind receives communication at one level while his or her unconscious mind processes other patterns of meaning from the words and develops related experiences (Erickson & Rossi, 1979). The therapeutic intention is to occupy, fixate, or disrupt the client's conscious frame of reference while generating an unconscious search for new or previously blocked meanings or solutions. Using metaphor, the therapist can:

- decrease the conscious resistance of the client;
- make or illustrate a point to the client;
- suggest solutions not previously considered by the client;
- seed ideas to which the therapist can later return; and
- reframe or redefine a problem for the client so the problem is placed in a different context with a different meaning (Zieg, 1980; Lankton, 2003/1980).

As a listener becomes increasingly engaged or absorbed in a story, there is a reduction in defensive mechanisms that customarily constrain the listener to sets of common (for them) experience. That is, listening to a story that symbolizes tenderness can lead a person who normally defends against sadness to weep. The concept of a novel experience may need slight elaboration. It pertains to experiences that are commonly excluded from the experiential set of the listener. While listening to an absorbing story, a client may, with relative ease, temporarily experience one or several specific experiences that, if therapeutically managed, can assist the listener in creating personal change.

The assistance in creating personal change comes about as clients reexamine perceptions or cognitions, emotions, or potential behaviors in light of a recognition that these new experiences, perceptions, or cognitions once thought to be alien actually are or can be a part of their own personality and experience. In general, it could be said that the usefulness of metaphor in therapy comes into play at any point in therapy where it is advisable or useful for clients to recognize that experiential resources lie within themselves rather than having to introject or incorporate them from an outside authority (including the therapist).

The outcome of metaphors *is determined by the experiences that are elicited* during the telling of the story. It can be assumed that the conscious mind of the listener will be engaged in the actual plot and development and of course conclusion of the story (if it is compelling). However, the unconscious outcome will be the result of elicited experiences evoked by the story. This is an important distinction to remember. The story is a vehicle for eliciting experiences, and that is often done with tangents taken from the storyline itself. If one thinks of the point of the story itself as the major therapeutic intervention, the client will only gain a cognitive understanding. The cognitive understanding is much like insight—and we know that insight does not change a person's behavior as much as a behavior change will lead to insight.

Simple Isomorphic Metaphors

Metaphors that can be described as isomorphic, and therefore parallel to the problem, are simple metaphors. They take the information from the client's life and match it one-for-one with the constructed story. That is, every significant noun in the original problem is matched with a noun in the story, and every significant verb in the problem is matched with a verb in the story. The relationship between the verbs and nouns is relatively obvious in that it is parallel to their relationship in the story.

The relationship between the problem and the story can be illustrated in the following example. Here we see that Joseph, who had a son named Paul, was in a car accident. The result of the accident was a serious injury of his son that took months to heal. As a result, Joseph feels a great deal of guilt. And as a result of the guilt, he remains jobless. He sought psychotherapy for assistance. A metaphor that could be built in an isomorphic fashion would be, for example, the one that follows. A building engineer who was in charge of construction crews was working on a building. Unexpectedly, the building collapsed and there were a great deal of injuries. One of the things that was "damaged" was the confidence of investors. All the investors abandoned the project. As a result, the building engineer felt helpless. As it turns out, his ability to seek and obtain employment was severely hampered by his feeling of helplessness, and he could not get any new investor contacts.

In graphic summary, would look like the following:

TABLE 1.1

Problem characteristics	Metaphor content
Joseph	Building engineer
Son Paul	Construction crew
Car	Building
Auto accident	Collapse of building
Serious injury	Investments lost
Guild	Helplessness
Joblessness	Can't secure a contract

This simple form of matching the problem to elements in the story can have a therapeutic usefulness as well as therapeutic limitations. Generally, it is easy to match the client situation with an imaginary or real story. However, the ending ought to be designed to be both reasonable with the story and retrieve useful therapeutic resources. It is most beneficial to formulate the ending that is the therapeutic goal before telling a story. These simple metaphors are also a useful form for delivering information to the client in a relative state of anonymity. That is, by the use of embedded quotes, or embedded commands, the therapist can illustrate dialogue within a simple metaphor. And, within that dialogue messages can be delivered to the client. For example, the therapist might say, "I had a client come see me this morning. And while he was on the elevator coming to my office, a total stranger looked at him and said, 'Get a job now and then you will start to feel better.'" Now, even without a sophisticated ending to this story, that client has gotten the instructional material that says something useful for the direction of therapy. It becomes thought provoking, to say the least.

A more sophisticated way to end isomorphic metaphors is to create a context in which the protagonist of the story retrieves useful resources to solve his problem. These resources will of course be parallel to the resources of the client.

Clinical observation suggests that clients make sense of the content of the metaphor because they apply their personal experience to the ambiguity in the story. Since this is the case, a metaphor that is parallel to the problem simply heightens their awareness of the problem. It is important for the therapist, therefore, to place emphasis upon the construction of the solution.

Since the important aspect of a metaphor is the construction of the solution, the entire metaphor can become parallel to the solution from the onset. Metaphors that are constructed in this manner are comparatively more sophisticated. These advanced metaphors are called complex goal-directed metaphors. The following brief outlines illustrate the major architecture of four different goal-directed metaphor protocols (Lankton & Lankton, 2007/1986).

Complex Goal-Directed Metaphor Protocols

A. Attitude change protocol
1. Describe a protagonist's behavior or perception so it exemplifies the maladaptive attitude. Bias the discussion of this belief to appear positive or desirable.
2. Describe another protagonist's behavior or perception so it exemplifies the *adaptive* attitude (the goal). Bias the discussion of this belief to appear negative or undesirable.
3. Reveal the *unexpected* outcome achieved by both protagonists that resulted from the beliefs they held and their related actions. Be sure the payoff received by the second protagonist is of value to the client listener.
B. Affect and emotion protocol
1. Establish a relationship between the protagonist and a person, place, or thing that involves emotion or affect (e.g., tenderness, anxiety, mastery, confusion, love, longing, etc.).
2. Detail *movement* in the relationship (e.g., moving with, moving toward, moving away, orbiting, etc.).
3. Focus on some of the physiological changes that coincide with the protagonist's emotion (be sure to overlap with the client's facial behavior and other identifiable bodily changes).

C. Behavior change protocol
   1. Illustrate the protagonist's observable behavior similar to the desired behavior to be acquired by the client. There is no need to mention motives. List about six specific observable behaviors.
   2. Detail the protagonist's internal attention or non-observable behavior that shows the protagonist to be congruent with his or her observable behavior.
   3. Change the setting within the story so as to provide an opportunity for repeating all the behavioral descriptions several (e.g., three) times.
D. Self-image thinking protocol
   1. Central self-image (CSI) construction
      a. Describe a protagonist who is seeing a reflection or picturing himself or herself accurately.
      b. Explain how the protagonist recalls and experiences several desired qualities (which may be resources retrieved earlier in the session).
      c. Describe how the original visual image of the self is altered in behaviorally specific ways consistent with each quality being experienced.
   2. Self-image scenarios process
      a. Using the story of the protagonist imaging his or her CSI as a device, describe imagined background details as follows.
      b. Introduce a positive, non-anxiety producing scene and people and describe the protagonist experiencing and thinking through behaviors in that scene (keeping the desired resources constant).
      c. Introduce other backgrounds and people in gradual successive approximations from the previous scenes to, eventually, the most difficult and contracted therapeutic goal.

The Ambiguous Aspect of Metaphor

Unlike directive and manipulative therapies that, through implication or connotation, tell clients how to perceive, think, feel, or behave, techniques of indirection allow clients to modify verbal input from the therapist and fit it to their own situation with a greater degree of relevance and with an element of ego-syntonic meaning. If clients are instructed to conduct themselves in a certain manner or say certain sentences to their spouse in directive couples therapy, these things may be ego-dystonic since they come from outside as implied or denoted by the therapist as something clients should or must do. However, when clients have determined for themselves a relevant meaning to a more ambiguous input from a therapist, they are acting upon perceptions, behaviors, or feelings that truly belong to them as a part of them.

Let's examine this ambiguous element more closely. The degree of ambiguity in a therapeutic story can be regulated by the teller so the story is more or less vague to the listener. Regardless of the degree of vagueness, listeners create their own relevant meaning in order to understand the story. This accounts for the ego-syntonic nature of the understanding and the lack of mere compliance by listeners. However, as the degree of vagueness increases, there is an exponential increase in the number of possible meanings that listeners can give to the story. It is assumed that listeners sorting through several possibilities at what has been determined to be thirty items per second (Erickson and Rossi, 1979, p. 18) become increasingly absorbed in weighing the best fit for these possible meanings. This ongoing process of weighing meaning has a number of therapeutic benefits:

- there is an increase in participation by listeners
- there is a heightened valuation in any meaning that is found by listeners as it has been made a deeper part of their own experience
- there is a depotentiation of normal, rigid ego controls while seeking a best fit
- there is an increase in the duration of time given to examining possible meanings

This last element, in fact, accounts for a therapeutic effect upon the client long after the therapy session has ended. Indeed, for a highly meaningful and yet extremely vague metaphoric story, listeners may continue to turn it over in their mind (from time to time) for years after the therapy session and do so for events that even years later parallel the original therapeutic learning incident. For this reason, the use of metaphor can be summarized as follows. It increases the relevance of therapy for clients and involves clients more highly in their own change process. It expands the usual limiting experience that has led to a stabilization of the presenting problem or dynamic and brought the person to therapy. It offers an engaging element of ambiguity that may continue to alert listeners to their therapeutic learnings for years after a therapy session. And it offers a wide range of potentially correct responses within the therapeutic limits.

Since indirect hypnotic language offers listeners the ability to apply a wide range or spectrum of potential understandings to what the therapist has said, there is a corresponding reduction in listener resistance. Any therapeutic modality that finds clients to be resistive, possibly due to the nature of the modality itself, will be able to take advantage of metaphoric stories providing those stories are constructed and shared in a manner that employs the necessary components of therapeutic change. Erickson once said:

I do certain things when I interview a family group, or a husband and wife, or a mother and son. People come for help, but they also come to be substantiated in their attitudes and they come to have face saved. I pay attention to this, and I'm on their side. Then I digress on a tangent that they can accept, but it leaves them teetering on the edge of expectation. They have to admit that my digression is all right, it's perfectly correct, but they didn't expect me to do it that way. It's an uncomfortable position to be teetering, and they want some solution of the matter that I had just brought to the edge of settlement. Since they want that solution, they are more likely to accept what I say. They are very eager for a decisive statement. If you gave the directive right away, they could take issue with it. But if you digress, they hope you will get back and they welcome a decisive statement from you. (Erickson, in Haley, 1973, p. 206)

ILLUSTRATION OF INDIRECT SUGGESTION LANGUAGE

Some of the most intriguing use of hypnotic language and perhaps the origins of indirect hypnotic language came from Erickson's work. It appears that *ambiguity* and *relevance* are the key factors to powerful therapeutic language. Clinically, it appears that the value of long-lasting hypnotic suggestion corresponds to the amount of ambiguity it conveys—while at the same time it appears to be personally relevant. The more ambiguity that can accompany an apparently relevant suggestion that creates a desired response, the longer and stronger that response will be. There is a limit to the amount of ambiguity each person can tolerate before a sense of relevance is impossible to maintain. Erickson appears to have learned this in his clinical work and supported it in the latter decades of his career. Indeed, ambiguity often allows language to seem more relevant. Consider the following examples.

Relaxation [direct suggestion]: "Let yourself relax. Let go of the tensions that you experience in your arms, allowing those muscles to become more and more relaxed . . . and let go of the tensions that you experience in your shoulders, allowing those muscles in your shoulders and back to become more and more relaxed . . . and let go of the tensions that you experience in your chest and belly and lower back . . . allowing those muscles to become more and more relaxed . . . and allow the muscles in your legs . . . to become more and more relaxed . . . your entire body . . . relaxing . . . until you feel limp and relaxed like an old rag doll."

Relaxation [indirect suggestion]: "I wonder if you know how it can feel . . . after a long day of physical activity when you've had a lot of things to do and you managed to accomplish everything and you get to the end of the day and you can finally let everything go and get some sleep? . . . everyone's had that experience . . . the conscious mind can't really appreciate how the unconscious can bring about an alteration that slows down the body . . . and the body for comfort maybe slowed it down for rejuvenation or for some other reason . . . and when a person gets ready for bed, slips between the sheets and feels those initial feelings . . . how cool and clean the sheets feel . . . what's the best word to describe that? . . . every child knows the feeling of comfort."

Suggesting eye closure [direct authoritarian suggestion]: "Now . . . your eyelids will become heavier . . . your eyelids are becoming heavier and heavier . . . so heavy that you cannot keep your eyes open . . . close them now."

Suggesting eye closure [indirect suggestion]: "Under what circumstances do the muscles of the face seem to support the eyelids? . . . they might become more and more relaxed or maybe just stop looking . . . I wonder which it will be in the case of each patient or each client . . . your conscious mind may wonder if your unconscious mind will actually close your eyes, or will it be the conscious mind that chooses to close your eyes so that you can let your unconscious mind wonder about a lot of things."

Creating Forms of Indirect Suggestion

The various forms of indirect suggestion and therapeutic binds might be seen as different specific vehicles for introducing ambiguity. That is to say, the different forms of indirect language are like specific different doorways into the mind. Ironically, the manner in which one can construct ambiguous indirect hypnotic language provides a great deal of therapeutic accountability. Using indirect language, the therapist can:

- introduce or illustrate a point to the client
- suggest solutions not previously considered by the client
- seed ideas to which the therapist can later return
- decrease the conscious mind resistance of the client
- reframe or redefine a problem for the client so the problem is placed in a different context with a different meaning
- retrieve and associate experience such as emotion, thought, perception, behavior, and expression.

In each case, just as in the case of metaphor, the ambiguity of the suggestion *requires that the client create personal meaning* out of the words. It is this act of creating personal meaning that gives indirect suggestion greater power and longer-lasting effect. The client actually will get the answer within their own experience and not comply to demands of the therapist.

Indirect suggestion can be an important part of accomplishing both the internal absorption and dissociation. The following section will give a brief glimpse as to what some of those forms of suggestion are and how they are formed. Six common forms of indirect suggestion and four common forms of therapeutic binds are representative of the large number of ways in which indirection can be codified.

Before beginning the illustrations of several forms of indirect suggestion and therapeutic binds, it is important to emphasize the following. These statements are intended to be formulated around a chosen therapeutic goal. In each case that chosen goal will be related to the next desired movement in the therapy. That is to say, if the client is seated and relaxed, the next desired goal might be to accomplish an induction with eye closure. On the other hand, if that has already been accomplished, the next desired therapeutic goal might be to help the client facilitate a sense of security or an intense memory of a desired experience. Regardless of the specific goal, the sentence structures that will be the vehicle for expressing that goal can be defined and delineated. This is not only useful for articulating the means by which hypnosis and therapy can be accomplished and taught, but also for carefully defining the procedures for the sake of future empirical research. The more carefully interpersonal communication can be specified, the more accurately empirical research can be carried out. Irrespective of these concerns, however, professional scholarship calls for a careful development and an earnest attempt to increase accountability of the therapeutic process. These forms of indirect suggestions and therapeutic binds, and more, were used by Erickson for both the induction of hypnosis and the process of psychotherapy during hypnosis and family therapy (Erickson & Rossi, 1980a, 1980b, & 1980c; Haley, 1963; Lankton & Lankton, 2008/1983; & Erickson 1980f).

Open-Ended Suggestions

Open-ended suggestions take the form of increasing the degree of ambiguity for any element in a sentence that would otherwise be a direct suggestion. In common social communication, it's usually an open-ended suggestion that introduces a topic. For example, an open-ended suggestion such as, "Everyone can find a way to record information that's important," could have been formed from the direct suggestion "Write this down." Since it's an open-ended suggestion, the degree of compliance from the client is irrelevant. Instead of telling the client what to do, it initiates the client's own search process for a discovery of what's relevant—if that happens to be writing down what's been said, then an exact fit between the otherwise unstated goal and what the client decides will have been made. But that's unusual. Open-ended suggestions are a prime example of how indirection is designed to be client centered and to facilitate helping clients discover their own understanding of what's relevant and useful to them, with the therapist still retaining an element of control, yet avoiding an authoritarian relationship.

Implication and Presupposition

The form of suggestion called presupposition is a simple type of implication. It can be a simple or complex presupposition, which then also states a desired goal. For example, a simple presupposition is, "*After* you write this down, we'll continue." This example uses a presupposition syntax (the word *after*), followed by the goal of taking notes by writing. Other simple presuppositions are: "*Since* this is the first time you've been in trance, close your eyes" and "*After* your trance is over, we'll do some talking about it" or "*One of the* first things you'll want to do in trance may be formulating a sense of comfort." In simple presupposition, the stated goal follows immediately after the presupposition syntax. It should be noted also that these suggestions are kept quite short. The reason for that is further speaking will begin to focus the client's attention elsewhere and become another form of suggestion I will discuss in a moment.

In each of those examples, simple presupposition was followed by a statement of the goal. The complex version involves the form called an implication. An implication requires that the speaker link two concepts together such that one relates to (e.g., causes) the other. And in addition, the concepts must have exact opposites—that is, the concept of "eyes open" has the opposite of "eyes closed." The concept of tense has the opposite of relaxed. So an implication that links "eyes open" and tension would be: "Keeping your eyes open can help you stay tense." Obviously the implication is that the listener will become relaxed when they close their eyes.

Questions or Statements That Focus Awareness

Indirect language suggestions that focus awareness can take the form of questions or statements. Statements such as, "I wonder if you'll be going into trance soon" or "I don't know if you've discovered how comfortable you are" have the effect of helping clients notice the portion of the sentence that highlights the goal and yet offers the sentence in a manner that seems to be rhetorical rather than strongly exclamatory. This form can also occur in questions such as, "Have you noticed how relaxed you are yet?" or "Do you think you'll begin thinking about the goal that we spoke of?" While these questions seem rhetorical, in order to consider them, the client must focus awareness as prescribed in the suggestion. In each of these examples a statement of the goal is presented following the question or observation.

Truism

Truisms state something that is essentially undeniable. Such sentences usually begin with phrases like, "All children" or "all people" or "in all cultures." For example, "All people have their own way of going into trance," "Every child uses imagination to think about ideas," "In every culture, people problem solve in various ways." In each of these examples, a truism is followed by statement of the desired goal.

All Possible Alternatives

Suggestions stating all possible alternatives can take several different forms, but have the common aspect of listing many different ways or times in which a stated goal can be reached or experienced. For example, "Your eyes may close suddenly or they may close slowly or you may close them and open them repeatedly, maybe you'll squint for some time, or it's possible that you'll have your eyes closed without realizing it and in some cases even have your eyes open and think that they're closed." Another example pertaining to relaxation could be, "You may relax systematically from your head to your feet or you may relax from your feet to your head, perhaps you'll discover some portions already relaxed and relax adjacent parts of your body, or it's possible that there will be a gradual relaxation all over your entire body at once, or possibly random limbs and muscle groups will relax in a more spontaneous manner or perhaps it will happen differently." In all possible alternative suggestions, it is advisable to have one of the alternatives state that the client will not do any of those on the list. This is because, in fact, you are trying to list all possible alternatives including the alternative that nothing of that nature will occur. In this form of suggestion, the therapist's list helps clients recognize that there are many ways the goal can be achieved and that they have a choice in how they personally express themselves. Therapists continue to establish an egalitarian relationship or client-centered relationship with the client rather than forcing an authoritarian and heightened compliant relationship.

Apposition of Opposites

This form of suggestion emphasizes that the occurrence of a desired goal may proceed paradoxically against some behavior that is generally seen as an opposite. For example, "The greater a degree of tension you have in your muscles, the more profoundly you may relax," "The longer you have been confused about the issue, the more rapidly an idea may come," or "The greater your uncertainty has been, the stronger your conviction may be." Clients can redirect and use energy previously devoted to avoiding or resisting to drive an equally strong, willful experience or behavior in the direction of their change. No reason or logic should be given for this paradox but rather clients should be allowed to discover for themselves how it becomes true for them. With indirect suggestion, the goal is not to make people behave in a particular way but rather to help stimulate their own thinking and experience in such a manner that they determine for themselves exactly what's relevant and how it's relevant for them.

Binds of Comparable Alternatives

The first of the four therapeutic binds is binds of comparable alternatives. In this type, two alternatives are provided so clients may choose which is best for them. In the process of making either choice, the actual desired goal is accomplished because it was presupposed by both choices. For example, "You may want to try these ideas in your family before you go to work; however, it may be best for you to try them after work." In this case, the act of trying the therapeutic material with the family exists for the client whether or not an attempt is made before or after work to implement the behavior. "You may go into trance by closing your eyes or you may wish to keep your eyes open" also facilitates going into trance regardless of the condition of the eyes.

Conscious/Unconscious Therapeutic Binds

The conscious/unconscious therapeutic bind takes a form that is somewhat like an algebra expression with an x and y variable, one for the conscious and one for the unconscious. The form of the sentence is: The conscious mind may do x as the unconscious mind does y. There are three things to consider about such a sentence. The first is what goes in place of the x. It is a good idea to place a word that refers to something that clients can verify with their conscious mind. Also some verb of mental activity such as *wonder, discover, know, investigate,* or *find* works very well in the position of x. This is especially true when there is only one specific therapeutic goal at that moment. What goes in place of the y in the formula is exactly what the goal is or some sub-portion of the goal at that moment. For example, if the goal happens to be to feel more comfortable spending time around one's new employer, the suggestion may state: "Your conscious mind may be surprised to discover how your unconscious will bring a feeling of relaxation around your new employer." If the goal is to relax in trance and recover a memory, the sentence could be formed as, "Your conscious mind may be relaxed while your unconscious investigates that memory." The third thing to consider with conscious/unconscious therapeutic binds is how the conscious and unconscious parts of the sentence are connected. There are a variety of causal links such as *and, as, since, while,* and *because* that can connect the two events. In general it is best to use a conjunction to link the two events together and avoid strong causal relationships.

Double Dissociative Conscious/Unconscious Therapeutic Binds

This form of bind is exactly the same as the previous one except that it accommodates two goals by duplicating and reversing variables on the conscious and unconscious as that phrase is repeated. An example of the formula is, "Your conscious mind may do x as your unconscious mind does y or, your conscious mind may do y as your unconscious mind does x." When x and y represent two different goals, they can or may become inexorably linked together by this type of verbal production. For example, if the goal is to feel comfortable and relaxed as you visualize interacting in a job interview, the sentence becomes, "Your conscious mind may be comfortable and relaxed as your unconscious rehearses how you will conduct yourself at the job interview or perhaps your conscious mind will rehearse how you will conduct yourself at the job interview while your unconscious mind is comfortable and relaxed."

Therapeutic bind is especially apparent in this sort of sentence. The client in trying to determine whether or not the first part or the second part of the sentence is the most true has, in fact, associated comfort and relaxation and visualizing the job interview. The only way to escape making the bind become true is to simply pay no attention to the actual content of the indirect suggestion used by the therapist—hence the understanding that these are therapeutic *binds*.

Pseudo Non-Sequitur Binds

The fourth form of bind is a pseudo-non-sequitur bind. I refer to them as "rephrasing binds" because a goal is stated and then renamed. A true non-sequitur question such as "Do you walk to school or carry your lunch?" may at first appear to be appropriately well formed as a question but actually bears no connection between the elements provided for choice and is therefore a non sequitur. In a pseudo-non-sequitur bind, two *apparently* different choices are provided for the client; however, the choices are simply the same option—spoken once and then reworded. This form differs from the bind of comparable alternatives because either choice is exactly the same choice. For example, "Do you think you'd like to go into a trance or would it be better to simply achieve an altered state appropriate for your learning today?" Another example is, "You could let all the muscles in your body go limp, or, if you prefer, to just relax completely."

USING INDIRECT SUGGESTIONS IN THE CONTEXT OF INDUCTION

No goal is likely to be reached by the utterance of a single suggestion but each goal can be addressed by using many of the different types of suggestion. This probably facilitates listeners processing the data with varying and different kinds of mental mechanisms. For example, presupposition, comparison, contrast, generalization, checking for fitness, choice, and so on. The differing forms of suggestions and binds require ferrying types of thought process. Therefore, by using various forms of suggestions and binds to restate therapeutic goals, the therapist enhances the possibility that clients will respond in a way that is meaningful to them. A brief example of an induction using these suggestions follows. The suggestions in the left column are labeled by the names of the suggestion appearing in the right column.

The suggestions in this brief induction are given as examples to facilitate an understanding of how trance induction might be developed using, primarily, indirection in a client-centered fashion in the clinical setting. It

TABLE 1.2

I don't know whether or not you've been in trance. After you reorient from trance we can discuss it. You can go into trance in your own way. Everyone goes into trance in a way that's unique for them.	statement to focus awareness presupposition truism truism direct suggestion ending with deletion
Just uncross your legs, put your arms at your side and begin.	pseudo-non-sequitur bind
You might develop an altered state that's appropriate for learning today or maybe develop a deep clinical trance. And you can do that rapidly, or suddenly, or you can go into trance and come out and go back in again, or you might simply gradually drift into a deep trance, or perhaps a medium trance, or nothing at all. You can go into trance with your eyes open or closed. But, go ahead and close them now. And let your conscious mind really wonder what the first thing your unconscious will do as you turn your attention inward. Did you wonder when you would go more deeply? You may find that your conscious mind is able to make some sense of things that your unconscious mind focuses on as you turn your attention inward or maybe your conscious mind, in turning your attention inward, will allow your unconscious mind to find some things that it can focus upon. Because, every human being has the ability to orient their experience toward that which is relevant. And the longer time you've spent in confusion wondering what to do, the more rapidly you may embrace the direction that seems right for you. Take your time to select memory of a time you felt most confident. And feel it now. The human mind has an amazing capability of applying previously learned experiences in new and useful ways.	suggestion covering all possible alternatives bind of comparable alternatives direct suggestion conscious/unconscious bind question to focus awareness with an embedded command double dissociative conscious/ unconscious bind open-ended suggestion acquisition of opposites direct suggestion direct suggestion open-ended suggestion

also illustrates how direct suggestion can be interspersed with indirect suggestion to facilitate the desired outcome. Greater detail and study and supervised training are always necessary for the appropriate and ethical use of suggestion in hypnosis and therapy.

Erickson believed that the depth of trance is less important than the relevance of the trance. He stated, "I find that one can do extensive and deep psychotherapy in the light trance as well as in the deeper medium trance. One merely needs to know how to talk to a patient in order to secure therapeutic results" (Erickson and Rossi, 1981, p. 3). The relevance of the trance will increase the degree of internal concentration and therefore increase the depth of trance. Each trance is individualized to the client, and scripted inductions should be avoided as much as possible. The state of internal absorption, the presence of some degree of ambiguity, and dissociation of the conscious mind establish a situation of communication with the client that is most conducive to helping that client focus upon and amplify various experiences.

RESEARCH

Overall, the Ericksonian tradition has been a lineage of "living wisdom" (like the passing on of martial arts skills) rather than a science. Most therapists realize the greatest amount of Ericksonian concepts and approaches when they are explained and demonstrated rather than from a critical examination of data supporting the theories and perspectives on hypnosis, the unconscious, and the nature of human experience. However, it is clear that much scientifically based research needs to be conducted to establish an empirically based Ericksonian body of knowledge.

The majority of articles appearing in refereed professional journals are publications of anecdotal case reports addressing many therapeutic venues and type of problems. These include brief therapy (Battino, 2007), utilization (Thomas, 2007; Akiyama, 2006), anxiety (Camino, Gibernau, & Araoz, 1999), depression (Young, 2006), post-natal well-being (Guse, Wissing, & Hartman, 2006), Candida (Edwards, 1999), family therapy (Crago, 1998), child therapy (Tennessen & Strand, 1998), solution focused (Santa, 1998), indirect suggestion (Fourie, 1997), and geriatric therapy (Gafner, 1997).

However, there is a paucity of empirical research showing what constitutes the effectiveness of an Ericksonian approach. Representative of what little exists ranges from therapeutic storytelling (Parker & Wampler, 2006), tailored and scripted inductions (Barabasz & Christensen, 2006), and visual recall in trance (Tamalonis & Mitchell, 1997) to research conducted on the effectiveness and subjective experience of hypnotic language and comparisons of direct and indirect suggestion (Alman & Carney, 1980). The following is a brief, but certainly not comprehensive, overview of some of that early research of indirect language in hypnosis.

Alman and Carney (1980), using audio-taped inductions of direct and indirect suggestions, compared male and female subjects on their responsiveness to posthypnotic suggestions. They reported that indirect suggestions were more successful in producing posthypnotic behavior than were direct suggestions.

McConkey (1984) used direct and indirect suggestions with real and simulated hypnotic subjects. Although all of the simulated subjects recognized the expectation for a positive hallucination, half of the real subjects responded to the indirect suggestions and half did not. He concluded that "indirection may not be the clinically important notion as much as the creation or existence of motivation where the overall suggestion is acceptable such as making the ideas congruent with the other aims and hopes of a patient" (p. 312).

Van Gorp, Meyer, and Dunbar (1985), in comparing direct and indirect suggestions for analgesia in the reduction of experimentally induced pain, found direct suggestion to be more effective reducing pain as measured by verbal self-reports and physiological measures. Stone and Lundy (1985) investigated the effectiveness of indirect and direct suggestions in eliciting body movements following suggestions. They reported that indirect suggestions were slightly more effective than direct suggestions in eliciting the target behaviors.

Mosher and Matthews (1985) investigated the claim by Lankton and Lankton (1983) that indirect hypnotic language created by embedding a series of metaphors will create a natural structure for amnesia for content presented in the middle of the metaphoric material. The authors compared treatment groups who received multiple embedded stories with indirect suggestion for amnesia with control groups who received multiple embedded metaphors without indirect suggestions for amnesia. They found support for the structural effect of embedding metaphors on amnesia.

Matthews, Bennett, Bean, and Gallagher (1985) compared subjects' responses on the Stanford Hypnotic Clinical Scale (Morgan & Hilgard, 1978) to subjects' responses on the same scale rewritten to include only indirect suggestions. They found no significant behavioral differences between the two scales. However, they did report that individuals who received the indirect suggestions perceived themselves to be more hypnotized than those who received the original Stanford Hypnotic Clinical Scale.

Nugent (1989a) attempted to show a causal connection between symptomatic improvement and the notion of "unconscious thinking without conscious awareness." In a series of seven independent case studies with a range of presenting problems (e.g., fear of injections, performance anxiety, claustrophobia), he used the same methodological procedure and treatment intervention of indirect suggestion language for change. A pretreatment baseline response and therapeutic change relative to the intervention were all systematically assessed. In all seven cases, each client reported a clear, sustained positive change with respect to the presenting problem using indirect lan-guage. Although the individual case study has certain methodological limita-tions, Nugent's use of seven independent cases with a carefully followed treatment protocol makes his conclusion of causality more convincing.

This brief overview of research results would appear to be mixed in sup-port of an indirect approach using suggestion, binds, and metaphor as com-pared with direct suggestion for many tasks. Direct hypnotic language was found more effective in treating pain in one study. However, indirect hyp-notic language was seen as most effective in eliciting movement behavior, producing trance depth, subjective experience of relevance, amnesia, and posthypnotic behaviors in other studies. And, when motivation was pres-ent, indirect suggestion was also seen as most effective for more difficult trance phenomena such as positive hallucination.

However, the reader should remember that for most of this research the tests were done with audio taping to standardize the intervention and that it was therefore not possible to tailor the suggestions (whether direct or indirect) and stories to the individual. A study by Barabasz and Christensen (2006) found that tailored inductions performed better than scripted inductions. As a result, the majority of these studies do not emphasize the importance of adapt-ing and using the unique responses of the individual throughout hypnosis.

Similarly, and perhaps more important, many of these tests were not designed in a context that attempted to address the relevant (growth) goals of individual subjects involved. Therefore, while the research gives us some idea, it does not represent a fully accurate picture of how a clinical client would experience the interventions when the hypnotic language is shaped and chosen for each individual.

Finally, these bits and pieces do not adequately address the entire course of treatment that would be considered Ericksonian in style. It is perhaps easier to discuss techniques than to discuss the subtle but more im-portant contributions of this overall approach. With an over-emphasis on technique, therapists have frequently been guilty of applying a technique without an adequate sense of how hypnotic language can develop within a natural interaction with clients.

CONCLUSION

As Haley notes, ". . . Dr. Erickson has a unique approach to psychotherapy which represents a major innovation in therapeutic technique" (Haley, 1967, p. 1). The therapeutic goal of an Ericksonian approach to hypnosis and therapy is to help clients concentrate upon and increase the use of desired experiential resources. This, in turn, is done to lead clients to change their relational patterns and bring a cessation to various presenting problems so they can live fuller and happier lives. Trance is a means of developing a state of heightened internal concentration for appropriate experiential resources that can be elicited and linked together. In turn, these gains must be conditioned to occur in specific life situations and during certain problem situations. Once that happens, a cure has been established.

Both of these aspects of heightened concentration and increased control of experience can be readily available when therapists use appropriate hypnotic language. An appropriate hypnotic language involves verbal and nonverbal communication that is understood as relevant and ambiguous to a certain degree. This *controlled elaboration of ambiguity* can be accomplished with utilization, reframing, indirect suggestions, therapeutic binds, simple and complex metaphor, and direct suggestion techniques.

Erickson's influence has grown from a seed to a forest over the last few decades. This is in large part due to his own tireless work and, after his death, the many dedicated faculty members who teach at professional training events sponsored by the Milton H. Erickson Foundation, Inc., the American Society of Clinical Hypnosis, the Society of Clinical and Experimental Hypnosis, the International Society of Hypnosis, and their subordinate events worldwide. Further, his work is advanced by the many books and professional papers written by these individuals.

At the time of this writing, a search of Amazon.com for Erickson's name lists 132 books. A search on the Internet today reveals 272,000 entries for Milton Erickson and 215,000 for Milton H. Erickson. There are currently 118 Erickson Institutes established worldwide for the further study and practice of Erickson's contributions to hypnosis, brief therapy, family therapy, and psychotherapy. Nevertheless, as with any talented innovator, the skill, perception, and capability of the originator seems to be a high-water mark in the field that is seldom achieved by subsequent generations of trainees. His clinically proven skill sets, like those of a complicated martial art, require careful study and practice, and time to replicate. His documented accomplishments with the skill sets will provide the motivation for years of material for future empirical research, evidence-based outcome studies, and the formulation of creative clinical applications. Finally, I want to caution readers, as did Jay Haley (Haley, 1993), on the care with which these powerful techniques should be exercised.

REFERENCES

Akiyama, K. (2006). Change of the client-therapist relationship through the utilization method. *Japanese Journal of Hypnosis*, *49* (2, Sept. 2006), 20–27.

Alman, B., & Carney, R. (1980). Consequences of direct and indirect suggestion on success of posthypnotic behavior. *American Journal of Clinical Hypnosis*, *23*, 112–118.

Araoz, D. (1982). *Hypnosis and sex therapy*. New York: Brunner/Mazel.

Bank, W. O. (1985). Hypnotic suggestion for the control of bleeding in the angiography suite. In Lankton, S. (Ed.), *Ericksonian monographs*, Number 1 (pp. 76–89). New York: Brunner/Mazel.

Bandler, R., & Grinder, R. (1975). *Patterns of the hypnotic techniques of Milton H. Erickson, M.D.* Cupertino, CA: Meta Publications.

Bandler, R., & Grinder, J. (1979). *Frogs into princes.* Moab, UT: Real People Press.

Barabasz, A., & Christensen, C. (2006). Age regression: Tailored versus scripted inductions. *American Journal of Clinical Hypnosis, 48*(4, Apr. 2006), 251–261.

Barber, T., Spanos, N., & Chaves, J. (1974). *Hypnotism, imagination and human potentialities.* New York: Pergamon.

Battino, R. (2007). Expectation: Principles and practice of very brief therapy. *Contemporary Hypnosis, 24*(1, Mar. 2007), 19–29.

Bekhterev, V. M. (1998). *Suggestion and its role in social life.* L. H. Strickland (Ed.) T. Dobreva-Martinova (Trans.). New Brunswick, NJ: Transaction Publishers.

Berne, E. (1972). *What do you say after you say hello?* New York: Grove.

Bowers, K. S. (1966). Hypnotic behavior: The differentiation of trance and demand characteristic variables. *Journal of Abnormal Psychology, 71,* 42–51.

Camino, A., Gibernau, M., & Araoz, D. (Trans). (1999). Ericksonian hypnosis: Applications in psychotherapy. *Australian Journal of Clinical Hypnotherapy and Hypnosis, 20*(1, Mar. 1999), 23–38.

Coe, W., & Scharcoff, J. (1985). An empirical evaluation of the neurolinguistic progamming model. *International Journal of Clinical and Experimental Hypnosis, 23,* 310–319.

Crago, H. (1998). The unconscious of the individual and the unconscious of the system. *Australian and New Zealand Journal of Family Therapy, 19*(2, Jun. 1998), iii–iv.

Dammann, C. (1982). "Family therapy: Erickson's contribution," in Zeig, J. (Ed.), *Ericksonian approaches to hypnosis and psychotherapy* (pp. 193–200). New York: Brunner/Mazel Publishers.

De Shazer, S. (1985). *Keys to solutions in brief therapy.* New York: W. W. Norton.

Dowd, E. T., & Hingst, A. G. (1983). Matching therapist's predicates: An in vivo test of effectiveness. *Perceptual Motor Skills, 57,* 207–210.

Dowd, E. T., & Pety, J. (1982). Effect of counselor predicate matching on perceived social influence and client satisfaction. *Journal of Counseling Psychology, 29,* 206–209.

Edwards, L. (1999). Self-hypnosis and psychological interventions for symptoms attributed to Candida and food intolerance. *Australian Journal of Clinical Hypnotherapy and Hypnosis, 20*(1, Mar. 1999), 1–12.

Erickson, B., & Keeney, B. (Eds.) (2006). *Milton H. Erickson, M.D.: An American healer.* Sedona, AZ: Ringing Rocks Press.

Erickson, M. (1980a). February man: Facilitating new identity in hypnotherapy. In E. L. Rossi (Ed.), *The collected papers of Milton H. Erickson on hypnosis: Vol. 4. Innovative hypnotherapy* (pp. 525–542). New York: Irvington.

Erickson, M. (1980b). Method employed to formulate a complex story for the induction of an experimental neurosis in a hypnotic subject. In E. L. Rossi (Ed.), *The collected papers of Milton H. Erickson on hypnosis: Vol. 3. Hypnotic investigation of psychodynamic processes* (pp, 336–55). New York: Irvington.

Erickson, M. (1980c). Special techniques of brief hypnotherapy. In E. L. Rossi (Ed.), *The collected papers of Milton H. Erickson on hypnosis: Vol. 4. Innovative hypnotherapy* (pp. 149–87). New York: Irvington.

Erickson, M. (1980d). Hypnosis: Its renaissance as a treatment modality. In E. L. Rossi (Ed.), *The collected papers of Milton H. Erickson on hypnosis: Vol. 4. Innovative hypnotherapy* (pp. 3–75). New York: Irvington.

Erickson, M. (1980e). Hypnotic Psychotherapy. In E. L. Rossi (Ed.), *The collected papers of Milton H. Erickson on hypnosis: Vol. 4. Innovative hypnotherapy* (pp. 35–48). New York: Irvington.

Erickson, M. (1980f). The confusion technique in hypnosis. In E. L. Rossi (Ed.), *The collected papers of Milton H. Erickson on hypnosis: Vol. 1. The nature of hypnosis and suggestion* (pp. 258–91). New York: Irvington.

Erickson, M. H. (1980g). *The collected papers of Milton H. Erickson on hypnosis: Vol. 1. The nature of hypnosis and suggestion.* E. L. Rossi (Ed.). New York: Irvington.

Erickson, M. H. (1980h). *The collected papers of Milton H. Erickson on hypnosis: Vol. 2. Hypnotic alteration of sensory, perceptual and psychophysical processes.* E. L. Rossi (Ed.). New York: Irvington.

Erickson, M. H. (1980i). *The collected papers of Milton H. Erickson on hypnosis: Vol. 3. Hypnotic investigation of psychodynamic processes.* E. L. Rossi (Ed.). New York: Irvington.

Erickson, M. H. (1980j). *The collected papers of Milton H. Erickson on hypnosis: Vol. 4. Innovative hypnotherapy.* E. L. Rossi (Ed.). New York: Irvington.

Erickson, M. H., & Rossi, E. (1979). *Hypnotherapy: An exploratory casebook.* New York: Irvington.

Erickson, M., & Rossi, E. (1980a). Varieties of double bind. In E. L. Rossi (Ed.), *The collected papers of Milton H. Erickson on hypnosis: Vol. 1. The nature of hypnosis and suggestion* (pp. 412–29). New York: Irvington.

Erickson, M., & Rossi, E. (1980b). Two level communication and the micro dynamics of trance and suggestion. In E. L. Rossi (Ed.), *The collected papers of Milton H. Erickson on hypnosis: Vol. 1. The nature of hypnosis and suggestion* (pp. 430–451). New York: Irvington.

Erickson, M., & Rossi, E. (1980c). Indirect forms of suggestion. In E. L. Rossi (Ed.), *The collected papers of Milton H. Erickson on hypnosis: Vol. 1. The nature of hypnosis and suggestion* (pp. 452–477). New York: Irvington.

Erickson, M., & Rossi, E. (1981). *Experiencing hypnosis: Therapeutic approaches to altered state.* New York: Irvington.

Erickson, M., & Rossi, E. (1989). *The February Man: Evolving consciousness and identity in hypnotherapy.* New York: Brunner/Mazel.

Erickson, M. & Rossi, E. (2008). An introduction to therapeutic hypnosis and suggestion. In Rossi, E., Erickson-Klein, R., & Rossi, K. (Eds.), *The collected works of Milton H. Erickson, Vol. 2, Basic hypnotic induction and suggestion* (pp. 1–8). Phoenix, AZ: The Milton H. Erickson Foundation Press.

Erickson, M. H., Rossi, E, & Rossi, S. (1976). *Hypnotic realities: The induction of clinical hypnosis and forms of indirect suggestion.* New York: Irvington.

Falzett, W. C. (1981). Matched vs. unmatched primary representational system and their relationship to perceived trustworthiness in a counseling analogue. *Journal of Counseling Psychology, 28,* 305–308.

Fisch, R. (1990). The broader implications of Milton H. Erickson's work. In Lankton, S. (Ed.), *Ericksonian monographs,* Number 7 (pp. 1–6). New York: Brunner/Mazel.

Fisch, R., Weakland, J., & Segal, L. (1982). *The tactics of change: Doing therapy briefly*. San Francisco: Jossey-Bass.

Fourie, D. (1997). Indirect suggestion in hypnosis: Theoretical and experimental issues. *Psychological Reports*, 80(3, Pt 2, June 1997), 1255–1266.

Gafner, G. (1997). Hypnotherapy with older adults. *Contemporary Hypnosis*, 14(1), 68–79.

Gill, M. M., & Brenman, M. (1959). *Hypnosis and related states: Psychoanalytic studies in regression*. New York: International Universities Press.

Gumm, W. B., Walder, M. K., & Day, H. D. (1982). Neurolinguistic programming: Method or myth? *Journal of Counseling Psychology*, 29, 327–330.

Guse, T., Wissing, M., & Hartman, W. (2006). A prenatal hypnotherapeutic program to enhance postnatal psychological wellbeing. *Australian Journal of Clinical & Experimental Hypnosis*, 34(1, May 2006), 27–40.

Haley, J. (1963). *Strategies of psychotherapy*. New York: Grune & Stratton.

Haley, J. (Ed.) (1967). *Advanced techniques of hypnosis and therapy: Selected papers of Milton H. Erickson, M.D.* New York: Grune & Stratton.

Haley, J. (1984). *Ordeal therapy*. New York: Jossey-Bass.

Haley, J. (Ed.) (1985a). *Conversations with Milton H. Erickson, M.D.: Volume 1, changing individuals*. New York: Triangle Press.

Haley, J. (Ed.) (1985b). *Conversations with Milton H. Erickson, M.D.: Volume 2, changing couples*. New York: Triangle Press.

Haley, J. (Ed.) (1985c). *Conversations with Milton H. Erickson, M.D.: Volume 3, changing families*. New York: Triangle Press.

Haley, J. (1973). *Uncommon therapy: The psychiatric techniques of Milton H. Erickson, M.D.* New York, Norton.

Haley, J. (1993). *Jay Haley on Milton H. Erickson*. New York: Brunner/Routledge.

Hammond, D. C. (1984). Myths about Erickson and Ericksonian hypnosis. *American Journal of Clinical Hypnosis*, 26, 236–245.

Hammond, D. C. (1988) Will the real Milton Erickson please stand up? *International Journal of Clinical and Experimental Hypnosis*, XXXVI(3), 173–181.

Henry, D. (1984). The neurolinguistic programming construct of the primary representational system: A multitrait multi-method validational study. University of Connecticut: *Unpublished master thesis*.

Hilgard, E. R. (1965) *Hypnotic susceptibility*. New York: Harcourt, Brace & World.

Hilgard, E. R. (1975) Hypnosis. *Annual Review of Psychology*, 26, 19–44.

Hilgard, E. R. (1966) Posthypnotic amnesia: Experiments and theory. *International Journal of Clinical and Experimental Hypnosis*, 14, 104–111.

Hilgard, E. R., Weitzenhoffer, A., Landes, J., & Moore, R. (1961). The distribution of susceptibility to hypnosis in student population: A study using the Stanford Hypnotic Susceptibility Scale. *Psychology Monographs*, 75(8), 1–22.

Kirsch, I. (1985). Response expectancy as a determinant of experience and behavior. *American Psychologist*, 40(11), 1189–1202.

Kirsch, I. (1990). *Changing expectations: A key to effective psychotherapy*. Pacific Grove, CA: Brooks Cole.

Laing, R. (1972). *Politics of the family and other essays*. New York: Vintage Books.

Laing, R. D. (1967). *The politics of experience*. New York: Ballantine Press.

Lankton, S. (1989). Motivating action with hypnotherapy for a client with a history of early family violence. In Lankton, S. and Zeig, J. (Eds.), *Ericksonian monographs*, Number 6 (pp. 43–61). New York: Brunner/Mazel.

Lankton, S. (2001). Ericksonian therapy. In R. Corsini (Ed.), *Handbook of innovative therapy* (pp. 194–205). New York: Wiley.

Lankton, S. (2003/1980). *Practical magic: The application of basic neurolinguistic programming to clinical psychotherapy.* New York: Crown Publishers.

Lankton, S. (2004). *Assembling Ericksonian therapy: The collected papers of Stephen Lankton.* Phoenix, AZ: Zeig/Tucker.

Lankton, C., & Lankton, S. (1989). *Tales of enchantment: Goal-oriented metaphors for adults and children in therapy.* New York: Brunner/Mazel.

Lankton, S., & Lankton, C. (1983). *The answer within: A clinical framework of Ericksonian hypnotherapy.* New York: Brunner/Mazel Publishers.

Lankton, S. & Lankton, C. (2007/1986). *Enchantment and intervention in family therapy: Using metaphors in family therapy.* New York: Crown Publishers.

Lankton, S., Lankton, C., & Matthews, W. (1991). Ericksonian family therapy. In Gurman, A. & Kniskern, D. (Eds.), *Handbook of family therapy.* New York: Brunner/Mazel.

Leary, T. (1957). *Interpersonal diagnosis of personality: A functional theory and methodology for personality evaluation.* New York: The Ronald Press.

Matthews, W. (1985) Ericksonian and Milan therapy: An intersection between circular questioning and therapeutic metaphor. *Journal of Strategic and Systemic Therapy, 3,* 16–26.

Matthews, W. (1985). A cybernetic model of Ericksonian hypnotherapy: One hand draws the other. In Lankton, S. (Ed.), *Ericksonian monographs*, Number 1 (pp. 42–60). New York: Brunner/Mazel.

Matthews, W., Bennett, H., Bean, W., & Gallagher, M. (1985). Indirect versus direct hypnotic suggestions—an initial investigation: A brief communication. *International Journal of Clinical and Experimental Hypnosis, XXXIII*(3), 219–223.

Matthews, W., & Dardeck, K. (1985). The use and construction of therapeutic metaphor. *American Mental Health Counselors Association Journal, 7,* 11–24.

Matthews, W., Kirsch, I., & Mosher, D. (1985). Double hypnotic induction: An initial empirical test. *Journal of Abnormal Psychology, 94*(1), 92–95.

Matthews, W., & Mosher, D. (1988). Direct and indirect hypnotic suggestion in a laboratory setting. *British Journal of Experimental and Clinical Hypnosis, 5*(2), 63–71.

Matthews, W., Lankton, S., & Lankton, C. (1996). The use of Ericksonian hypnotherapy in the case of Ellen. In S. J. Lynn, I. R. Kirsch, and J. W. Rhue (Eds.), *Casebook of clinical hypnosis* (pp. 365–91). Washington, DC: American Psychological Association.

McConkey, K. (1984). The impact of indirect suggestion. *International Journal of Clinical and Experimental Hypnosis, 32,* 307–314.

Morgan, A., & Hilgard, J. (1978). The Stanford hypnotic susceptibility scale for adults. *American Journal of Clinical Hypnosis, 21,* 148–169.

Mosher, D., & Matthews, W. (1985). Multiple embedded metaphor and structured amnesia. Paper presented at the American Psychological Association meeting, San Diego, CA.

Nugent, W. (1989a). Evidence concerning the causal effect of an Ericksonian hypnotic intervention. In Lankton, S. (Ed.), *Ericksonian monographs*, Number 5 (pp. 68–85). New York: Brunner/Mazel.

Nugent, W. (1989b). In Lankton, S. (Ed.), A multiple baseline investigation of an Ericksonian hypnotic approach. *Ericksonian monographs*, Number 5 (pp. 69–85). New York: Brunner/Mazel.

O'Hanlon, W. (1987). *Taproots*. New York: Norton Publishers.

Orne, M. (1959). The nature of hypnosis: Artifact and essence. *Journal of Abnormal and Social Psychology, 58*, 277–299.

Parker, T., & Wampler, K. (2006). The use of therapeutic storytelling. *Journal of Marital & Family Therapy, 2*(Apr. 2006), 155–166.

Parsons-Fein, J. (2004). *Loving in the here and now*. New York: Penguin.

Ritterman, M. (1983). *Using hypnosis in family therapy*. San Francisco: Jossey-Bass.

Rossi, E., & Ryan, M. (Eds.) (1985). *Life reframing in hypnosis*. New York: Irvington.

Rossi, E., Ryan, M., & Sharp, F. (Eds.) (1983). *Healing in hypnosis by Milton H. Erickson*. New York: Irvington.

Santa, R., Jr. (1998). What do you do after asking the miracle question in solution-focused therapy? *Family Therapy, 25*(3), 189–195.

Stone, J. A., & Lundy, R. M. (1985). Behavioral compliance with direct and indirect body movement suggestions. *Journal of Abnormal Psychology, 3*, 256–263.

Tamalonis, A., & Mitchell, J. (1997). Empirical comparison of Ericksonian and traditional hypnotic procedures. *Australian Journal of Clinical Hypnotherapy and Hypnosis, 18*(1, Mar. 1997), 5–16.

Tennessen, J., & Strand, D. (1998). A comparative analysis of directed sandplay therapy and principles of Ericksonian psychology. *The Arts in Psychotherapy, 25*(2), 109–114.

Thomas, F. (2007). Scout's honor. *Journal of Family Psychotherapy, 18*(3), 2007, 85–89.

Ueshiba, M. (1991). *Budo*. Tokyo: Kodansha International.

Van Gorp, W. G., Meyer, R. G., & Dunbar, K. D. (1985) The efficacy of direct versus indirect hypnotic induction techniques on reduction of experimental pain. *International Journal of Clinical and Experimental Hypnosis, 4*, 319–328.

Watts, A. (1957). *The way of zen*. New York: Vintage Press.

Watzlawick, P., Weakland, J., & Fisch R. (1974). *Change*. New York: W. W. Norton & Co.

Weakland, J., Fisch, R., Watzlawick, P., & Bodin, A. (1974). Brief therapy: Focused problem resolution. *Family Process, 13*, 141–168.

Weeks, J. R., & Lynn, S. J. (1990). Hypnosis, suggestion type and subjective experience: The order effects hypothesis revisited. *International Journal of Clinical and Experimental Hypnosis, 38*, 95–101.

Weitzenhoffer, A. M. (1957). *General techniques of hypnotism*. New York: Grune & Stratton.

Weitzenhoffer, A. M., & Hilgard, E. R. (1963) *Stanford hypnotic susceptibility scale, Form C*. Palo Alto, CA: Consulting Psychologists Press.

Yapko, M. D. (1982). The effect of matching primary representational system predicates on hypnotic relaxation. *American Journal of Clinical Hypnosis, 23*, 169–175.

Young, G. (2006). Hypnotically-facilitated eclectic psychotherapeutic treatment of depression: A case study. *Australian Journal of Clinical Hypnotherapy and Hypnosis, 27*(1, Fall 2006), 1–13.

Zeig, J. (Ed. with commentary). (1980). *A teaching seminar with Milton H. Erickson*. New York: Brunner/Mazel.

Zeig, J. (Ed.). (1982). *Ericksonian approaches to hypnosis and psychotherapy*. New York: Brunner/Mazel.

Zeig, J., & Lankton, S. (1988). *Developing the Ericksonian therapy: state of the art*. New York: Brunner/Mazel.

Chapter 2

Ego Psychology Techniques in Hypnotherapy

Arreed Franz Barabasz

To paste a coping skill on the surface of an injured person is to further remove that person emotionally from the "self."
(Watkins & Barabasz, 2008; Watkins & Watkins, 1997)

The human personality is not a unity, although it is usually experienced as such. Our personalities are separated into various segments. Unique entities serve different purposes. This is the central premise of ego state therapy.

The state that is overt and conscious at a particular time is the executive state. Those states that are not executive may or may not be aware of what is going on at a conscious level. Conflicts among states take up considerable energy, often forcing the individual into withdrawn, defensive postures. A person, such as in the case of Mathew below, will not be at peace with himself until the conflicts are resolved.
(Watkins & Barabasz, 2008)

Mathew is in a new relationship with Emma. He sees Emma playing with a child. He feels and believes, "This is the woman for me. I love her and I want to spend the rest of my life with her." Later in the same day she criticizes him about his job as a plumber. He feels defensive and thinks, "What did I ever see in this woman? How can I get out of this relationship?" These responses may sound extreme, but they are not unusual, and it is not unusual for a person to bounce among several ego states in the process of making a major decision (one state may be in favor, one may be against, and another indifferent). In one moment on one day Mathew may "know" he wants Emma as his partner, and in another moment he may know "he does not." In this example, Mathew has an ego state that loves and dreams of a family. It is a soft, caring part of him, and when he sees the woman he cares about playing with a child his "loving/caring" ego state becomes executive. While in this state, Mathew is capable of feeling very positive and interested in Emma. These are honest feelings. It is Mathew who is feeling them. It is Mathew's "loving/caring" part. Later, when Emma criticized his job, another part of Mathew is energized to become executive (comes out). Mathew's "defensive, don't pick on me" ego state becomes executive. This is not a loving, caring part of Mathew, and probably can't even feel love. Its role is to protect, by creating a shell and withdrawing from the attacker. While in this state, Mathew cannot imagine life with Emma. This too is a part of Mathew, just as valid and needed as the other.

                                                              (Emmerson, 2003, p. 2)

As shown by Mathew, in the previous case, an ego state is "an organized system of behavior and experience whose elements are bound together by a common principle." However, each state is separated from other states by a boundary that is *"more or less permeable"* (Watkins & Watkins, 1997, p. 25). Each is distinguished by a particular role, mood, and mental function, which when conscious [executive] assumes the person's identity. Ego states start as defensive coping mechanisms and when repeated develop into compartmentalized sections of the personality (Emmerson, 2003, p. 3). They may also be created by a single incident of trauma such as an auto accident, rape, or even the first day of kindergarten. Ego states maintain their own memories and communicate with other ego states to a greater or lesser degree. Unlike alters in multiple personalities in those with dissociative identity disorder (DID), ego states are a part of normal personalities.

THE EVOLUTION OF EGO STATE THERAPY

Hypnosis pioneer Pierre Janet (1907) seems to have been the first to describe those covert personality segments with which we will concern ourselves within ego state theory and therapy. Janet's focus was on the study of true multiple personalities (dissociative identity disorder) and was probably the first to use the term *dissociation* to describe systems of ideas that were split off, thus not in association with other ideas within the personality. He also implied that these personality patterns can exist subconsciously in normal functioning individuals even though not overt and available to conscious observation and experience.

As one of the first psychoanalysts to deviate from pure Freudian doctrine, Carl Jung (1969) also recognized well-established covert structures within the "collective" or unconscious. These were termed "archetypes." More transient groups of unconscious ideas clustered together were referred to as a "complex." Although the terminology varies from that of Janet as well as our own, both Jung's concepts of a personality "complex" as well as the more structured "archetypes" he is best known for refer to personality segments that are organized into unconscious patterns.

Paul Federn (1952a) was the first to systematically apply the concept of ego states to provide a psychodynamic understanding of human behaviors. His disciple Eduardo Weiss (1960) translated his papers, published them, and extended many of their implications. Neither Federn nor Weiss ever seemed to fully realize the great significance of ego states in their treatment procedures, nor did they seem to understand that an alternative theoretical formulation was needed to comprehend its potential as a new sophisticated form of hypnoanalysis. This endeavor became one of John G. Watkins's greatest contributions to the science and practice of psychotherapy (AFB).

John G. Watkins was the first to recognize that Federn's theory was entirely limited to only ego-energized items. Watkins modified the conceptualization and developed the theory of ego states with his wife Helen Huth Watkins. This new theory includes ego-energized *and* object-energized elements. Thus, when they have become organized together in a coherent pattern, the ego state may represent an age of a relationship in the individual's life, which may have been developed to cope with a certain situation (Barabasz & Watkins, 2005; Watkins, 1978; Watkins & Watkins, 1979, 1981, 1982, 1986, 1997).

Let's say your patient was severely punished as a five year old. Becoming quiet, saying little, and withdrawing passive aggressively was a way of handling the situation. Such coping patterns seemed to also work in later life. So when in "trouble with an authority figure" the adult now finds the five-year-old ego state returning no matter how short sighted, present oriented, and ultimately self-defeating it may be. As Marlene Hunter (2004, p. 88) points out, those with borderline personality disorder "still cope the way they did when they were 5 years old."

Thus, our conceptualization of an ego state is one that includes both ego and object energized elements that are encompassed within a common principle, a collection of subject and object items that belong together in some way and that are included within a common boundary that is more or less permeable. By "permeable" we mean that it is accessible by the conscious and sometimes, but not always, in subconscious communication with other co-existing ego states.

When one of these states is invested with a substantial quantity of ego energy it becomes the "self in the here and now." We say that it is *executive* and it experiences the other states, if it is aware of them all, as "he," "she," or "it" since they are primarily invested with object energy. As ego and object energies flow from one state to another, the behaviors and experiences of the individual change, and we may assign the diagnosis of Dissociative Identity Disorder (DID; Multiple Personality Disorder). Defined in this way, ego states subsume what we call "multiple personalities" but also include other clusters of mental functions, which may or may not reach consciousness and directly change behavior.

THE MOST SIGNIFICANT HUMAN EXPERIENCE: SUBJECT-OBJECT

My leg is me. My arm is me. My thought is me, or is it, if I am hallucinating? Subject-object, what is within my "self," and what is not, is perhaps the most significant area of human experience.

Perceptions refer to mental images and sensations, which are normally elicited by objects outside the body. But a stone in the stomach and infection in the blood are also "objects." An arm is normally considered as "subject," part of me. But if it is paralyzed and devoid of feeling and movement, then it, too, becomes an object. An idea, a concept is normally subject—it is "my" thought. But a hallucination is an idea, which is perceived as coming from the outside. The hallucination is not perceived as part of me, therefore, it is perceived as object.

Clearly then, the body cannot be the criterion for distinguishing between object and subject. The entity which does so discriminate is our essence, "the self." That which is perceived as outside "myself" whether it is within the body or not is "object." That which is *experienced*, as within "my self," hence, part of "the me," is subject. The "self" and not the body is the distinguishing agent, and the difference is judged by our *feeling of selfness* when we are aware of it.

THE SELF

The self and what constitutes it has been the subject of numerous theories as well as scientific controversies. Freud (1933) postulated a state of "primary narcissism," an inherent condition in the original child. Later, he viewed the ego as a structure within the mind, which was equated with the self. This was apparent in his topographic conceptualization of the mind when one looks at it as originally written in German. The ego structure was represented as the *selbst*, literally translated into English as the "self." Hartmann (1958) regarded the ego, hence the self, as not only an inherent structure, but partially determined by the impact of the veridical world on the developing infant. Other object-relations analysts, such as Winnicott (1965) saw the self and its feeling of self-existence as coming about as the mother, who acts like a mirror, reflects back to the child his or her own experience and gestures. The child then believes that "when I look, I am seen, so I exist." When the mother resonates to the child's needs, the latter becomes aware of them. This awareness then slowly evolves into this sense of self. It is the "me" inside, sometimes working and serious, sometimes at play, sometimes in pleasure and others in pain. Mahler (1972) emphasized the maternal role in developing the child's self through a separation-individuation process by which he or she comes to know himself or herself. As the child interacts with mother, the child separates himself or herself to develop a unique identity and sense of selfness.

Similarly, Hartmann (1958) considered the "self" as an object representation or experiential construct, but Kernberg (1976) extended this formulation to reserve the term *self* to "the sum-total of self-representations." By this he apparently meant that certain experiences, feelings, and images were endowed with self-feeling that interacted with other images and sensations that were felt as "not me," but were also represented within the mind. This interaction is embedded within the ego and constitutes "the self."

I (J.G.W.) proposed a similar view (Watkins, 1978, ch. 6) that "existence" occurred only when an object, "a not-me," impacted a subject, "a me." This is consistent with Fairbairn's conceptualization (see Guntrip, 1961) that ego and object are inseparable. An object is not significant (e.g., does not exist to its perceiver) unless it has some ego energy in contact with it.

The classical theory developed by Freud in its original form posited that the individual was born with innate drives, sexual and aggressive, and that it was in the satisfaction or frustration of these that personality structure and neurotic conflicts developed. Analysts operating from this basic assumption became known as "the drive model analysts." These theorists and psychotherapists were considered the original members of the relational school who increasingly emphasized the role of interpersonal relationships as a basis for shaping all human development. As the relational branch of object relations theory developed, opposition to the drive/libido theory grew. Harry Stack Sullivan (1968) highlighted the interpersonal dimension arguing that Freud's theory could be better understood on the basis of interpersonal processes. Sullivan's elaborate conceptualization of psychopathology emphasized a person's behaviors that are intended to minimize or avoid anxiety that was rooted in dreaded thoughts of rejection and derogation by parents, others, and eventually oneself. Sullivan explained that particular aspects of the child, such as crying or whining, result in parental rejection or ridicule (e.g., telling a boy to "stop acting like a girl"). Integrating that these parts represent an anxiety arousing "bad self," these aspects are "split off or disowned." What Sullivan overlooked is that although they may be split off they are not killed off; disowning by repression assures they remain as covert ego states that continue to affect behavior in less-than-ideal ways given that their overt expression has been denied. Our ego state conceptualization suggests such split-off unexpressed child fixed ego states are likely to become malevolent. However, Sullivan did recognize that the child develops coping mechanisms to preclude being subjected to anxiety-arousing rejection again (Teyber, 2000, p. 6). Unfortunately, in adulthood these responses become characterological as the child now grown to adult size anticipates that new experiences with others will repeat the relational patterns of the past.

Eventually, patients' childlike attempts to contain their bad aspects will lead to frustration. The self-effacing patient will not win approval of everyone they need, the aloof patient will be forced by situational demands to compete with others, and the expansive (histrionic) patient will not always succeed at manipulating others to defer to their demands. When such a student receives anything less than 100 percent approval from an instructor or mentor, they will feel completely defeated and overreact with great drama toward a significant person and may engage in storytelling in an effort to seek attention from others. Therapists who fail to recognize this expression of an often repressed ego state (the "narcissistic wound" in Kohut's [1977] interpersonal process terms) will question this overreaction and provide a rational appraisal of the situation. This attempt at reality grounding might well result in a transference reaction toward the therapist who has missed entirely the deeper meaning to the client coming from the frustrated childish ego state. The therapist must grasp the patient's point of view that this seemingly minor rejection indicates once again for the patient that no matter how great their efforts they cannot get it right. Rather than reject the ego state that is expressing such desperation, the therapist should reflect compassion for the burden of perfectionism that the client has suffered from since childhood. This resonant understanding will strengthen the therapeutic alliance and create, especially with the aid of hypnosis, a safe place for the patient to explore collaboration of their ego states.

Kohut (1971, 1977) departed most from "drive theory." In his *Psychology of the Self* (1977), Kohut assigned the classical functions of ego, super-ego, and id to the self. He hypothesized that this entity was developed by the infant's internalization of "self-objects," meaning the significant people in the child's world, usually his or her parents. Through their empathic responses to his or her needs, they provided the experiences necessary for the development of the child's "self." This is an extension of Mahler's concepts, but unlike her, Kohut broke more definitely with the drive theory approach since he perceived the self as almost entirely a product of interpersonal relations. Kohut felt that the self expresses a need for contact with others as its basic motivational apparatus rather than sexual or aggressive drives.

Because of loyalty to Freud, and their own wish to be identified with the body of classical psychoanalysis, the object-relation theorists and to a lesser extent the interpersonal process theorists kept trying to reconcile their new concepts, derived from clinical experience with classical drive theory (Greenberg & Mitchell, 1983). All of these practitioners were inhibited, at least to some degree, in proposing concepts of personality development, which departed too widely from accepted theories. Innovative psychological theories that deviated too radically from Freud's, such as Alfred Adler's

(1948), Carl Jung's (1916), and Otto Rank's (1952) had all resulted in the past with their author being rejected from membership within classic psycho-analysis. Kohut's views, which were probably the most progressive of the object relation theorists, were most likely more closely aligned than the other three to the earlier views of Paul Federn, who was a friend and close associate of Sigmund Freud.

PAUL FEDERN'S EGO PSYCHOLOGY

Federn was one of the first to join Freud's group and developed innova-tive techniques for treating psychosis. As early as 1927, Paul Federn had proposed many of the concepts advocated later by the object relations and interpersonal process theorists. His work was almost completely ignored in the controversies between drive model and relations model theorists as he remained all but unreferenced by those credited with the development of object relations theory. One gets the impression that they never read Federn, and it remained to Eduardo Weiss (who was analyzed by Federn and trained by Freud) to publish an English compilation of Federn's papers. The ignorance of Federn's contributions may stem from three primary problems. First, Federn wrote in what almost any upper-level graduate stu-dent would view as complex, long-winded, German sentences. Weiss, who was John G. Watkins's analyst, once said to J. G. W., "Federn is very diffi-cult to understand. That is why I had to write an introduction to his book to explain him." At that time, J. G. W. was in analysis with Weiss. J. G. W. noted, "I had not acquired the courage to say, 'But Dr. Weiss your writ-ings are also hard to understand'" (Watkins & Barabasz, 2008).

Another reason may have been that Federn used alternative terminol-ogy to refer to psychoanalytic structures and processes that were then cur-rently in normal usage. Federn himself was not fully aware of the extent to which his view departed from Freud's. At any rate, his theories have not been widely read nor understood by the few that have attempted their reading. Federn's theories, however, provide a foundation for Ego-State Therapy as a unified theory, which integrated the use of hypnosis to dra-matically speed psychoanalytic processes and its extensions. After more than a quarter century of development by John and Helen Watkins as the primary formulators of the theory and therapy, Ego State Therapy is now considered established. The first "World Congress of Ego State Therapy" was held March 20–23, 2003, in Bad Orb, Germany, with the recognition and sponsorship of both the German and European Hypnosis Societies. Ego State Theory was again a central focus of the European Society of Hypnosis Congress held in Gozo, Malta, September 18–23, 2005, and most recently at the International Tagung Ego – State Therapy: Hypnosis, Trauma and Psychotherapy, Kathmandu, Nepal, May 4–8, 2008, and in Pokhara, Nepal, May 12–14, 2008.

EGO STATE THEORY

As is well known, Freud based much of his theory on the displacements of a single energy, libido, which originated in the id. He later hypothesized the need for two variants of libido: narcissistic libido and object libido. Yet this still represented only two different allocations of the same energy source rather than two different kinds of energy. Hartmann originally (1955) referred to "a primary ego energy," which was not derived from instinctual libidinal energy. Later, Jacobsen (1964) supported an initial state of undifferentiated energy, which then acquires libidinal or aggressive qualities. Kohut (1971), while attempting to appear loyal to Freud's drive theory, proposed that libidinal energy could be divided into two separate and independent "realms," including narcissistic libido and object libido. All of the psychodynamic object-relations and interpersonal process theorists recognized that Freud's single energy theory, libido, was not adequate to account for the phenomena, which they observed in their patients. Their tortured writings show numerous efforts to force these phenomena into a single energy (libido) mold.

Federn had broken with that position much earlier and had clearly formulated a two-energy theory that resolved many of the conflicts in understanding psychodynamic processes and thus provided a rationale for more effective therapeutic interventions (see Federn, 1952a). It also provided a rationale for hypnotherapy and hypnoanalysis, a consequence not envisioned by either Federn or Weiss.

EGO AND OBJECT ENERGY

Federn hypothesized different energies: "ego energy and object energy." The term *libido*, as formulated by Freud, meant an instinctual sexual energy emanating from the id. It was also an object energy, since it could be displaced to various objects such as the patient's mother, who then became an object of erotic interest further extended by Jung (1966), who regarded it as life energy to differentiate it from that of purely sexual energy. To avoid the confusion, let us follow both Federn's and Weiss's later terminology and use only "ego energy and object energy."

Energy can be defined as an investment of a quantum of energy to activate a process. A motor is "energized" with electricity and then runs. Ego energy is the energy that cathects or activates the ego. It is the energy of the self. In fact, it is the self. Ego energy is what you are, it is the "you" in you. Self is an energy, an organic, life energy, not a compilation of feelings, thoughts behaviors, and so forth. Ego energy has but one basic quality, the feeling of selfness, of me-ness. If an arm is invested or energized with this ego energy, then I experience it as "my" arm. If a thought is invested or activated with ego energy, then I experience it as "my" thought. It has become part of "the me," and, therefore, I regard it as within "myself." By calling it "ego energy" and not "ego libido," we will no longer confuse it with the instinctual, sexual, and object energy.

Federn's second energy was "object energy." It is qualitatively very different, being a nonorganic energy, much like electricity, radiation, and so on. It has but one basic quality. Like ego energy, it can activate or make a process go, but any process or body part object energized is not experienced as "me." It is sensed or perceived as an object, hence, outside "my" self. Patients suffering from borderline personality disorder (BPD) ascribe only such object energy to other humans in their life space. To them, people serve a purpose but do not have selfness.

Kohut and other object relations–interpersonal process theorists were apparently unaware of Federn's work and did not seem prepared to challenge Freud's drive theory to the point of recognizing that the concept of a single kind of energy called libido had to be eliminated to bring the theoretical structure to fruition in the treatment of patients. Instead, Kohut and the others continued to modify the concept of the manner of cathecting by a single energy, which determined whether a representation became a "true object" or a "self object." It seemed that at some level Kohut recognized the need for a two-energy approach but could never bring himself to such a conceptualization.

Federn's concept of two different kinds of energy directly challenged Freud's basic views regarding a single, unitary "libido." As such, it was ignored by many psychoanalysts until the advent of Ego State Therapy.

Neither ego energy nor object energy should be equated in any way with consciousness. If my arm has been hypnotically anesthetized, paralyzed that is, and removed from my self-control, its ego energy has been removed (dissociated). The arm is now experienced by me as an "it," an external object and entirely outside of "myself." If the paralysis is hypnotically removed and the "feeling of selfness" restored, that is because we have invested it again with ego energy. From this perspective, hypnosis is clearly the modality of choice for directing the various displacements of ego energies and object energies.

Existence is impact between object and subject, so consciousness in ego state theory is an economic matter. When the impact of an object-energized element on an ego-energized boundary exceeds a certain magnitude, we become aware, hence, conscious of it. This depends both on how highly energized the object is and how highly energized the ego boundary is. We can become aware of strongly energized (energized objects) even if the ego boundary is lightly energized and the impact of a low-energized object may become conscious if the receiving ego boundary is highly energized. If you stroke my hand lightly, I may not feel anything. If you slap it strongly, I become aware of the touch. As you develop a highly tuned listening, ego boundary, hence, a sensitive third ear (Reik, 1948), you may become quite aware of an unconscious and symbolic communication from your patient, which the more obtuse practitioner will completely miss.

Introjection and identification depend on the allocation of object or ego energies. When I introject an outside person—perhaps my father—I have erected a mental image, a replica or representation of my father based on my perceptions of him. This introject is an object because at this time it is invested with object energy. If my father was a critical person, at the time that I introjected him, I will feel (perhaps unconsciously) the lash of his criticism within which I may simply experience as depression. It, a "not-me," is critically and harmfully impacting "the me." There may also be an introject of a partner, or friend. These are always persons who are, or least have been, meaningful at some time in your patient's life. The patient is frequently astounded at the emotions they experience while an introject is executive, yet by such experiencing in the first person the patient develops a better understanding of that introject and their limitations.

Introjects are not ego states. They are not part of the patient's personality, yet, they can be treated in much the same way as an ego state is and perhaps most importantly they can change to bring greater health to the patient's adaptability and functioning in life. Introjects can be scary, abusive, and threatening, or kind and helpful. As Emmerson (2003, p. 12) points out, when the significant person in the person's life was benevolent, an introject will then also be benevolent. However, an introject that had been internalized as cold and scary may, through ego state negotiation, become warm and caring. Thus, as we will discuss later, it is frequently helpful for ego states to be encouraged in therapy to express themselves as introjects. The hypnotized client can express feelings toward the malevolent introject by being encouraged to speak to those interjected emotions and told, "What you did to me was wrong!"

No doubt you will have at one time heard the phrase, "If you can't beat 'em, join 'em." Psychodynamically, we call it "identification with the aggressor." For example, let us say you are employing ego state therapy to treat a borderline personality disorder. You know the disorder was developed in your patient due to abandonment of a significant other, usually a parent. The child fixates at the age at which the abandonment occurred and internalizes the concept that they deserve to be abandoned as they must have been bad. Accordingly, to escape from the internal criticism, which as in the previous case may have been expressed as depression, I may "identify" with my father. Hence, a common choice in borderlines is in choosing a series of psychologically or physically abusive, controlling significant others. What happens here is that I remove the object from this representation and invest it instead with ego energy. I infuse the representation with the feeling of self-ness. The introject is no longer a "not-me" object but instead has become part of "the me." I experience it within myself. I am no longer depressed by my father's introjected criticisms; but I am now critical of my own children.

The content of the "introject" has not been changed. It has now become an "identofact," a part of "my" self. I have become like my father, and the neighbors say, "He is just like his father." In so identifying with such a significant other, your patient becomes sicker and less able to adapt in any overall sense, thus, mature functioning and healthy adaptation is precluded. In object relations terminology we might note that what had been an "object representation" has now become a "self representation." (At first, the patient sees the serious problems in the individual and then becomes just like that individual.) This same maneuver is possible with hypnotic intervention through hypnotic suggestion. Ego and object energies can be manipulated therapeutically to the benefit of the patient (subject-object techniques are reviewed in Barabasz and Watkins, 2005, pp. 49 and 177, and elsewhere in that volume).

The object relations and interpersonal process theorists are sometimes difficult to understand because they often confuse introjects and identifications. Kohut (1977), for example, appears to define the term of what earlier analysts called introjects of significant others, which at first are objects but later are changed into identifications. He believed that such entities are necessary even in adaptive mature adults.

In Federn's Ego Psychology, the term *self-object* is contradictory. A representation of a significant other constructed within the individual will either be activated by object energy, like an introject, as previously discussed, or energized by ego energy, like an identification. The child's "merger" with such "self-objects" may be gradual; a "representation" cannot be both "self" and "object" at the same time since this is determined by the quality or nature of the activating energy. It cannot be experienced as "me" and as "not me" at the same time.

HYPNOSIS AND ENERGIES

Hypnosis emerges as the key modality for moving and changing of energies when formulating treatment plans for your patients on the basis of object and subject energies. One hypnotically suggests to a patient that he or she is now able to move a hysterically paralyzed limb—this may happen because ego energy has now been invested in it, changing it from object to subject, hence, bringing it within the self and back to the patient's voluntary control.

Similarly, by hypnotically moving more object energies into a circumscribed repressed memory, it becomes strong enough to impact the ego boundary so as to render it conscious. Energies can also move into an object or process whenever we simply pay attention to it.

Federn did not employ hypnosis in his treatment, yet he foreshadowed its use in Ego State Therapy. Eduardo Weiss, in his introduction to Federn's book (Federn, 1952a, p. 15), wrote, "Ego states of earlier ages do not disappear, but are only repressed. In hypnosis, a former ego state containing the corresponding emotional dispositions, memories, and urges can be re-awakened in the individual." This was a rather profound statement for that era.

If a hypnotized participant's hand is made to wag up and down (Barabasz & Watkins, 2005) without conscious control, we have simply removed its ego energy. It is anesthetized and apparently not within the control of the amused subject. Its movement is now object energized. The wagging can become voluntary only if it is ego energized. Hypnosis thus becomes a very powerful therapeutic modality for altering ego and object energy changes within our patients.

PSYCHOSES AND EGO ENERGIES

Federn's most significant contribution stemming from his two-energy theory was in the understanding of psychotic symptoms and the psychotherapeutic treatment of the psychoses (see Federn, 1952a, chs. 6–12). Federn characterized a hallucination as a pseudoperception. The schizophrenic actually sees, hears, or otherwise senses something that does not really exist in the outer world. To the psychologically ill patient these perceptions appear to be quite real, as can be well verified by the clinician who tries to persuade the client otherwise. Yet, the stimuli from these pseudoperceptions arise from within the patient—that is, the patient's own inner cognitions. They represent ideas that are normally experienced as subject—that is, as stemming from one's self. The psychotic, however, experiences them as object and similar to other outside objects that he or she sees, hears, or otherwise senses.

How can thoughts be turned into perceptions? Federn hypothesized that psychotic patients sense the contents of their delusions and hallucinations as real because they originate from repressed mental stimuli that entered consciousness without obtaining ego energy, not because of faulty reality testing as graduate students are frequently taught and many in our field assume. The problem is in the weakness of the ego boundary. Like a geographical boundary, such as that between two countries that is inadequately patrolled by border guards, citizens can be mistaken for aliens and vice versa. In the psychotic, the inability to test reality adequately results from an energy deficiency—a lack of sufficient ego energy to patrol the ego boundaries, where the differentiation must be made for normal adaptation to the outside world. Federn's approach was intended to help the patient build more ego energy. That, of course, is precisely what we do with relationships, supportive therapy, exercise, and so forth. In the implementation of such an approach, Federn often (please consider the era of the mid-1900s) used a nurse, a mother-surrogate, who could provide the nurturing relationship normally received from one's mother (Schwing, 1954).

The mother figure is critically important because her nurturing in developing self-identity and stable object representations, which Federn and Schwing had been emphasizing, has currently begun to receive more attention. The significance of mothers as "transitional objects" in the development of self structures in infants has been increasingly recognized (Baker, 1981; Barabasz & Christensen; 2006 Christensen, Barabasz, & Barabasz, 2009).

Baker (1981), Copeland (1986), and Murray-Jobsis (1984) have employed many of these same concepts in treating psychotics within the hypnotic modality with remarkable positive and lasting outcomes.

REALITY A REALITY B

Now what was happening here is that Federn, and especially his disciple Weiss (1960), stressed the distinction between reality testing and the sensing of reality. We "sense" reality as something outside our self whenever an object-energized item impacts an ego boundary. However, to "test" reality we need to use our eyes, ears, and body and note that the sensed object moves its relative position accordingly. The schizophrenic, for example, fails to take this action, relying instead entirely on his or her weakened ego boundary in a desperate attempt to distinguish real from unreal, thoughts from perceptions. Federn reported that there is a felt difference between an impact of an object on the "inside" of the ego's boundary and its "outside," that which interacts with the external world. If this is also true, there would have to be a change in the magnitude of the impact. The psychotic then would be able to experience this "reality" of his or her reported experience when it is explained to the patient that there are in actuality two kinds of reality, "reality A" and "reality B." The idea here is to enlist the patient's cooperation rather than the patient's antagonism when being confronted with reality as if they were being accused of "lying."

What might said to the patient is, "When you see me here I want you to label that 'reality A.' When you see or hear those people who are persecuting you, I want you to please call that 'reality B.' Now 'reality A' is a kind of experience you can share with others around you because they, too, are aware of 'reality A.' However, 'reality B' is a private reality, which they cannot share. If you talk to them about 'reality B' they will think you are crazy! Please do this, when you describe to me any experience, tell me, at least for now, whether it is 'reality A' or 'reality B.'"

Testing this remarkable intervention with numerous psychotic patients, Federn concluded that psychotic patients could, indeed, distinguish between reality A and reality B even though both were experienced as real. By teaching these patients to make this discrimination, he was exercising, strengthening, and re-energizing their ego boundaries. In time, these patients made this distinction. By not reinforcing reality B, the hallucinated "reality" was de-energized. Reality B was then returned to the world of nocturnal dreams, wherein lie the consciously inactive "hallucinations" of normal people. By reducing the energy in reality B, its impact with self-boundaries became lower than the threshold necessary to become conscious.

By positing a two-energy system, Federn provided a new rationale to explain many psychological processes that cannot be satisfactorily accounted for by Freud's one-energy (libido) system. For example, if a thought of my dead mother crosses my mind and reaches consciousness, but is activated with object energy, I will experience it as a perception of my dead mother. I will "see" her. And, if I report this perception as real, others will say I am psychotic and hallucinating.

Years ago, John G. Watkins was trying to explain the mechanism of projection to a paranoid patient. As we all know, that is usually a futile task. Much to his surprise, the patient smiled and said, "Well doctor, if you are trying to tell me that those men who persecuted me were a product of my own imagination, you don' t have to. I arrived at that conclusion my self over the weekend." In utter amazement, Watkins spent some time evaluating him before accepting that his delusions and hallucinations had disappeared. The patient's own unconscious hatreds externalized into a perception of "men out there" who were persecuting him, had been de-energized of object energy, and were now energized with ego-energy. He experienced them as his thoughts and not his perceptions. The critical point I am trying to make here is that a one-energy system would not give us an adequate explanatory rationale even though psychodynamically we are still unaware of just what caused this energy shift.

Psychologists and psychoanalysts frequently confuse subject and object. Thus, an introject is supposed to be an internal object. Yet, analytic writers portray a patient as "introjecting" another person when they describe that individual as acting and talking like the other person. The image of the other, when internalized, is at first invested with object energy. That is why it is an internal object. An introject is like that submarine sandwich you ate one late evening that lies in the stomach ready to resurface at midnight. It is within the self but not part of it, ingested but not digested.

For the individual to act and talk spontaneously like any other, the object energy must be withdrawn and ego energized. In object-relations theories, we would simply say that the object representation has changed into a self-representation. Then we no longer have an introject; we have an identofact. The internalized has become part of "the me."

For example, a teenage girl "in love" imitates the behavior of her boyfriend, eating what he eats and regressing to earlier behaviors by acting as immaturely as he does. This action is at first an introject of that same-age immature boyfriend's behaviors. Eating like him, behaving like him, and taking on his views are simply internal representations of the boyfriend, copied but not part of her own self. However, in the course of time, it may become automatic. The behaviors have become egotized—that is, invested with ego energy. It is now part of her own self. Her same-aged but now more mature girlfriends watch her behaving like her boyfriend does and are amazed. If he lacks future goal directed plans, she too loses focus; if he is opinionated, bitter, or selfish, she is too. She has identified with her boy-friend. An identification with a previously introjected other may be minimal or significant, depending on how much of the other's physical attributes and or psychological behavior, as in the present example, is taken over. As Watkins (1978a) points out, an introject is the result of the process of introjection, and a new term is needed to distinguish between the process of identification and the result of that process. Consider our use of the word *identification* when referring to the process, and the term *identofact* to indicate the internal, ego-energized image that has been created by identifi-cation. The girl described herein has changed the introject, and object repre-sentation, of her "boyfriend" into an identofact, a self-representation. This distinction between what is subject (ego-energized) and what is not self (object-energized) in physical and psychological processes is crucial. The movement from one to the other is fundamental to the practice of ego state therapy, as well as many other treatment approaches.

PERSONALITY DEVELOPMENT: INTEGRATION AND DIFFERENTIATION

Personality develops through two basic processes, integration and differen-tiation. By integration, a child learns to put concepts together, such as cow and horse to build more complex units called animals. By differentiation, he or she separates general concepts into more specific meanings, such as discrim-inating between a cat and a rabbit. Both processes are normal and adaptive.

Normal differentiation permits us to experience one set of behaviors at a party Saturday night and another at the office Monday morning. When this separating or differentiating process becomes excessive and maladap-tive, we call it dissociative identity disorder.

When we differentiate two items, both of which are consciously in mind, we can compare them and note their differences. In dissociation, the two items are so separated from each other that comparison is not pos-sible, since only one is within consciousness at any given time. Both differ-entiation and dissociation involve the psychological separating of two entities, but differentiation is lesser in degree, generally adaptive, and con-sidered to be normal. Dissociation, on the other hand, is considered to be pathological. It may be more immediately adaptive to cope with the stress of a specific situation, but often at the future expense of greater maladap-tiveness. Differentiation and dissociation may be considered as simply resulting from different degrees of the separating process.

EGO STATES

To understand the nature of ego states one must consider their origin. Most frequently, they were first created when the individual was quite young. They think concretely like a child. Because of the emergence of primary process thinking as produced by hypnotic age regression (Barabasz & Christensen, 2006; Christensen, Barabasz & Barabasz, 2008), adult logic, therefore, may not reach them, even though they often talk in an adult voice. It is as if they were frozen in time. Covert ego states, unlike the alters in a true multiple personality (DID), require hypnosis for their activation. But, if they first originated when the patient was a child, then one should think of them like a small girl who is dressed up in her mother's clothes and pretending to be an adult. The ability to think concretely like a child has been lost by the majority of adults, and thus we are at a disadvantage in dealing with child ego states, especially when they are not so clearly differentiated as true multiple-personality-like alters. States that were created during the patient's teens will still think like a teenager, rejecting and suspicious of grown-ups and very defensive of their own (pseudo) independence; they do not want to be told what is right or what they ought to do. This characteristic is illustrated in the case excerpts (see Watkins & Barabasz, 2008).

When working therapeutically with child and adolescent states, one should conceptualize to whom one is talking and conduct the interaction accordingly. The clinician or counselor who resonates well will have the greatest probability of success.

Be mindful that a child ego state was developed to adapt to the conditions of days gone by, not today. Its attempts to function today result in maladaptive behaviors (short-sighted present rather than future-oriented actions). As one inquires and secures information about the time and circumstances when an ego state first appeared, one's approach can be modified accordingly, even though one is confronted ostensibly with a full-grown adult. This modification can be done, without embarrassment, by the use of hypnosis. The psychotherapist interacts as one would with a child when the patient is hypnotized.

Bear in mind that an ego state was most likely developed to enhance the individual's ability to adapt and cope with a specific problem or situation in the past. Thus, one ego state may have taken over the overt, executive position when dealing with parents, another on the playground, another when dealing with a significant other, and yet another when participating in a sporting event, and so on.

In the case of dissociative identity disorder, which is manifested by the presence of true multiple personality alters, the specific situation is usually some very severe trauma such as child abuse or traumatic abandonment. The ego state forms to help in dissociating the pain from the primary alter or to make it easier for the major personality to deal with an abuser (controller) without inviting retaliation. It is to be expected that these specific ego states will be reactivated in the transferences of the present, such as to teachers, employers, supervisors, mentors, colleagues, and, of course, therapists (Watkins & Barabasz, 2008).

A common trait is that once created, ego states are highly motivated to protect and continue their existence. The clinician who tries to eliminate (kill off) a maladaptive state will find to his or her dismay that the entity probably does not want to disappear, but that one's intervention has now created an internal enemy who resists therapeutic intervention. Part-persons seek to protect their existence, as do whole-persons. This tendency also has important implications in the treatment of dissociative identity–disordered patients. Perhaps the most important point to remember is that it is much easier to modify the motivations of malevolent and maladaptive ego states and their behavior constructively than to attempt to eliminate them.

Persistence in existence is to understand that the original ego state came into being to protect and facilitate the adaptation of the primary person. It remained because it had a certain amount of success. It was positively reinforced, first for coming into existence, and then for continuing its presence. It makes no difference whatsoever that now its efforts may be contra productive to the person. The earlier adaptations, which are now maladaptive, will hold precedence.

First, we must familiarize ourselves with the differences in the environment of the patient's past and that of the present. We cannot generally induce a state to change into an adaptive stance toward current adult problems when the treating counselor or clinician does not understand its earlier struggles. Recognition of these traits is essential in the planning and conduct of effective therapeutic maneuvers such as abreactions (Barabasz, 2008a,b,c).

When working with ego states, the internal equilibrium of the patient will change in such a way that a new ego state, or one that has been long dormant, will be energized and make itself known. This state may first manifest itself by slight changes in posture, mannerism, or voice pitch.

Using the explanatory value of Federn's two-energy theory makes it easier to understand. The nature of the past problems helps us to determine the creation and energies of the various states. The adaptational needs of the present must be met with the appropriate dispositions of object and ego energies assisted by an understanding and accepting therapist. Hypnosis is the key modality that facilitates this allocation of subject and object energies. This treatment goal can be reached from a variety of orientations according to the clinician's primary training including behavioral, psychoanalytic, cognitive-behavioral, Rogersian, and existential therapies. Any such approach constitutes ego state therapy when the goal is appropriate dispositions of object and ego energies.

Ego states that are cognitively dissonant or have contradictory goals often develop conflicts with each other. When they are energized and have rigid, impermeable boundaries, multiple personalities (DID) may result. However, many such conflicts appear between ego states only covertly, and these are often manifested by anxiety, depression, or any number of neurotic, maladaptive, and childlike behaviors.

Ego states may be large, encompassing broad areas of behavior and experience, or they may be small including very specific and limited reactions. They may also overlap. For example, a six-year-old child ego state and a "reaction to father" ego state both speak the English language. They can range from minor mood shifts to true overt multiple personalities, the difference being the permeability of their separating boundaries.

EGO STATE BOUNDARIES: THE DIFFERENTIATION-DISSOCIATION CONTINUUM

Psychological processes do not exist on an either-or basis. Anxiety, depression, immaturity, and so forth all lie on a continuum with lesser or greater degrees of intensity. So it is with differentiation-dissociation. On one end of the continuum, the boundaries are so permeable that they are almost nonexistent. The individual's behavior is very much the same from time to time. The difference that does occur is generally adaptive, and we call it normal differentiation. As the ego state boundaries become increasingly rigid, intrapersonal communication is impeded so that behavior becomes less and less adaptive. When we approach the end of the continuum, the boundaries are very rigid and impermeable, the behavior is maladaptive, and we call it "dissociation." At this extreme end of the continuum, the various ego states no longer interact or communicate with one another and the individual suffers from a true multiple personality (dissociative identity disorder) if more than one becomes energized enough to assume the overt executive position temporarily.

In between these extremes lies a body of ego states that may act like "covert" multiple personalities, but which do not spontaneously become overt. However, they can be activated hypnotically.

The various states are conscious of the existence of one another but refer to the others as "he, she" or "it," and not as "me." This position on the differentiation-dissociation continuum represents a bordering (almost true) multiple personality and is not to be confused with the diagnosis of borderline personality disorder. The in-between ego states, because of the lesser degree of rigidity in the semipermeable boundaries, retain partial communication, interaction, and sharing of content. In general, they remain covert and do not spontaneously appear overtly, but they can be activated into the executive position by hypnosis. In this region, a conflict between the states may be manifested by headaches, anxiety, withdrawal, passive aggressive, and other maladaptive behaviors, such as are found in the neuroses and in the psychophysiologic disorders. It is in this area where the most productive contributions of ego state concepts to psychotherapy have occurred. We are, therefore, concerned with a general principle of personality formation in which the dispositions of the activating energies and the impermeability of the boundaries separating the organized ego-state patterns have resulted in relatively discreet personality segments that may alternate in assuming the executive position, experienced as "the self" in "the here and now." The extreme form of this separating process, as noted before, can result in true dissociative identity disorders.

For some time, true multiples were considered to be extremely rare. However, as recognized in the *Diagnostic and Statistical Manual of Mental Disorders-IV* (APA, 1994) and in the more recent text revised (TR) edition, many reports of cases meeting full diagnostic criteria are now being presented. The disorder is still uncommon but it can no longer be considered rare. For example, borderline multiples are frequently misdiagnosed as borderline personality disorders. This is fairly common and particularly prevalent among females, and may be due to the higher frequency of abuse of females as children as well as gender-specific maladaptations to abandonment.

CHARACTERISTICS OF EGO STATES AND DISSOCIATIVE IDENTITY DISORDER

Ego states should be regarded as part-persons. Except in the case of true multiple personality (DID), they do not normally appear overtly unless hypnotically activated. There is far too much evidence to the contrary to impute to them simply as therapist-created artifacts since they often differ widely from therapist expectations. Some act like complete "persons." Others appear to be very limited personality fragments, perhaps created for a specific defensive purpose. They may have quite differing interests, purposes, and values, even as do the various alters in a true dissociative identity–disordered personality. Obviously then it is not surprising to find them often in intra-personal conflict with one another, creating tension, anxiety, psychosomatic symptoms, the desire for flight, and other maladaptive behaviors. As one ego state put it, "I make her eat because if she is over-weight men (who are dangerous) will not be attracted to her." Covert ego state conflicts may create headaches just like the quarreling of multiple personality alters who struggle to emerge and take over executive control of the body.

EGO STATE THERAPY

Ego state therapy is the utilization of individual, family, and group therapy techniques for the resolution of conflicts between the different ego states that constitute a "family of self" within a single individual (Watkins & Watkins, 1997, p. 35). Therapy involves a kind of internal diplomacy that may employ any of the cognitive-behavioral, psychoanalytic, Rogersian, or humanistic techniques of treatment but almost always uses hypnosis. These techniques are directed toward the part-persons represented by the ego states and not toward the whole individual. While it is possible to practice ego state therapy in the conscious condition (Emmerson, 2006), the use of hypnosis is the method of choice for most practitioners. This is because ego states, unlike true dissociative identity disorder (DID) alters, do not usually become overt spontaneously. Most of the time they require hypnotic activation. Through hypnosis we can focus on one segment of personality and temporarily ablate or dissociate away other parts. In fact, since hypnosis is itself a form of dissociation, it is not surprising to find that good hypnotic participants often manifest covert ego state segments in their personalities even though they are not mentally ill. Hypnosis offers access to levels of personality that in classical psychoanalysis require much, much longer periods of time to contact. Since ego state therapy is an approach involving inter-part communication and diplomacy, hypnosis generally becomes an essential for practicing it when the states are covert.

At times an ego state may be exerting an influence as "object" on the primary individual—in which case we might say, "I would like to talk to that part" (we don't use the term *ego state* with the patient) of Mary Anne who has been compelling her to overeat (or who knows about her overeating). A communication back from such a "part" commonly is the result. The content of this "part" is often at considerable variance with the therapist's expectations, contradicting the notion that ego states are only artifacts created to please the therapist (a common argument posed by those who incompletely understand ego state therapy).

Only being "part-persons," ego states often think concretely like a child and must be communicated with accordingly. Sometimes ego states appear during sleep or in hypnosis-like dream figures. The same general strategies and tactics used in treating DID patients apply when working with the more covert ego states except that they must be preceded by a hypnotic induction.

EFFICACY RESEARCH

Much of the recognition of the efficacy of ego state therapy has been based on clinical experience rather than controlled research as evidenced by the acceptance of this approach at the First World Congress on Ego State Therapy held in Bad Orb, Germany, in 2003, and most recently in Kathmandu, Nepal, in 2008. Nonetheless, controlled research, although still in its infancy (Frederick, 2005), thus far indicates that ego state therapy is effective in assisting clients with both psychological and somatic symptoms. Using a time series analysis as the experimental procedure, Emmerson and Farmer (1996) found that women with menstrual migraines were able to experience not only a significant reduction in headaches, but also a reduction in depression and anger. This occurred following a four-week treatment with ego state therapy. The monthly average number of days with migraine went from 12.2 to only 2.5. Consistent with this decline in headaches was a statistically significant decline in levels of depression and anger. The ego states text (Watkins & Watkins, 1997) reports on 42 clients who had received ego state therapy for a median of only 11 hours total treatment and those who had received other types of therapy with a median of 145 hours. Twenty-four clients said ego state therapy met their expectations, while only seven clients said the other therapies met their expectations. Gainer (1993) also reported very positive effects of ego state therapy. When trauma held by a child ego state was processed, there was complete remission of Reflex Sympathetic Dystrophy (Ginandes, in press).

EGO STATES AND HIDDEN OBSERVERS

Little more than a quarter of a century ago, Ernest R. Hilgard was demonstrating hypnotic deafness before a class of students at Stanford University. As Barabasz and Watkins (2005) explain, to dissociate something one must first be aware of it at some level, or as Martin Orne's trance logic conceptualization would dictate, "you have to hear it or see it before its presence can be negatively hallucinated away." Given that understanding, let us get back to Hilgard's fascinating demonstration. As he was about to invoke hypnotic deafness, a student in his class asked whether some part of the apparently deaf subject might be aware of what was going on. Hilgard then said to the hypnotized subject, "although you are hypnotically deaf, perhaps there is some part of you that is hearing my voice and processing the information. If there is I should like the index finger to rise as a sign that this is the case." Much to Hilgard's surprise, the finger lifted! Later, he discovered that individuals similarly reported being aware of pain (but without its sensation) in a hypnotically anesthetized hand. Hilgard ascribed this phenomenon to a cognitive structural system, which he called "the hidden observer."

Watkins and Watkins (1979–1980) conducted a set of experiments in which they activated hidden observers in former ego state therapy patients using the same procedures and verbalizations employed by Hilgard in his studies, repeating with both hypnotic deafness and hypnotic analgesia. What emerged were various ego states with which they had dealt in treatment over a year earlier. They hypothesized that hidden observers and ego states are, therefore, the same *class* of phenomena.

To conclude this discussion, let us note the differences between Federn's original conception of ego states and Watkins's view of them. To Federn, the ego remained a constant. Different contents could pass in and out if it by being ego-energized, which were then organized by the ego into the ego states. When an ego state was de-energized of self-energy, it retained its organization and continuous existence as an object representation. An ego state consisted only of self-energized items. In our view (Watkins &

Barabasz, 2008), the self consists of pure ego-energy, not contents, such as motivations, affects, ideas, and so forth. This energy is not the energy of the self, *it is* the self.

When this ego energy passes into contents, these are then experienced as part of the self; in other words, they are experienced as "me." The movement is on the part of the self energy as it passes into and out of various organized behavior and experience patterns we call ego states. Such a state may contain both object *and* self representations, which on repression, removed from consciousness, still retain their respective and relative structures. Thus, this ego state, whether self or object-energized, is the unit to be dealt with in therapy. It takes on the character of the major amount of energy within it, ego or object, and is experienced by the individual as such, "the me" or less frequently as the "it." Looking once again at the figure showing the differentiation-dissociation continuum, it is worth noting that hidden observers and other partially separated personality segments exist as ego states within the middle range.

EGO STATE THERAPY TREATMENT

The ego state therapy session typically resembles family therapy in that one member speaks, another is asked to respond, and an exchange of communications begins. Sometimes it is necessary to call on specific states to come out and speak. At other times they will emerge spontaneously so long as the hypnotic state has been adequately established. Sometimes no one will abdicate if pressed too hard, and another will appear. The important point is that the therapist thinks of it as talking to a multiplicity and not a unity. There is a single body in view but you are dealing with a family. What one says to one ego state may well be heard by others who can take offense and oppose one's treatment efforts.

The counselor or clinician operates like a group therapist. Any therapeutic maneuver, such as reflection, ventilation, desensitization, abreaction, free association, interpretation, reinforcement (approval), clarification, and so forth that is part of your armamentarium may be employed. These can be used within the basic theoretical orientation that you have been trained in. However, they are to be applied with the use of hypnosis and to the various personality segments rather than to the patient viewed as a unity.

Sometimes the awareness of what has been done with an ego state may be brought to the attention of the conscious person. At other times, efforts will be made to strengthen some of the more constructive ego states. Occasionally, an ego state can be found that may serve as an assistant therapist, consulting with the clinician about strategy, advising of the effects of earlier maneuvers, and helping in planning future steps. We (Watkins & Barabasz, 2008) have taught ego states, who at first were destructive, to become constructive. It is our job to try at all times to discover and meet the needs of each ego state. Where they are conflicting, negotiation and compromise are indicated. Your role as a psychotherapist is frequently that of a communicator and a mediator between the clashing states. For example, "George" (a teenager ego state) was asked, "Would you be willing to do your homework during the week if "father" (a parental ego state) doesn't bug you about playing on the weekends?"

Remember that ego states, like dissociative identity disorder alters, originated for defensive adaptive purposes during the person's critical developmental years and/or in response to trauma such as faced by soldiers in the Iraq wars, so they may no longer now be adaptive for the individual. As they were developed when the individual was a child and/or for immediate survival defense mechanisms, they do not serve well for normal functioning adults. It is, therefore, unwise to eliminate "bad" ego states. Rather, one can avoid much resistance if you treat all the ego states with the utmost courtesy and respect, secure their cooperation, try to meet their needs, and play the role of a good friend to each. Attempts to eliminate a state mobilizes much resistance that can sabotage treatment.

SUMMARY

Ego state therapy was derived from the study of multiple personalities and experiments with normal, hypnotized subjects within the general theoretical structure of hypnoanalysis. Hilgard's "hidden observers" and the theories of Paul Federn served as an origin for its conceptual structure. However, we (Barabasz & Watkins, 2008) have elaborated on its original formulations and altered them in certain significant areas based on our experimental studies and clinical experiences.

It is essential to recognize that the "separating function" in the formation of personality structure, like almost all psychological processes, exists on a continuum ranging from normal, adaptive differentiations through defensive operations to maladaptive dissociation as exemplified in true dissociative identity disorder.

Ego state therapy may use any of the directive, cognitive-behavioral, analytic, or humanistic approaches in treatment. But it applies these to personality segments, that is, part-persons, and not to the entire individual. Generally, it does so with the use of hypnosis since covert ego states do not typically appear spontaneously without having been hypnotically activated.

The orientation here is hypnoanalytic ego state therapy. However, a therapist with a different theoretical orientation might prefer to practice a hypnocognitive ego state therapy, applying his or her interventions to part-persons (ego states) rather than to the entire individual.

Ego state therapy is a very potent treatment procedure because it focuses on the specific areas of the personality that are most relevant to the presenting problem. This tactical advantage is valuable not only in dealing with the occasional true multiple personality, but extending to the vast array of neurotic, psychosomatic, and behavioral disorders ranging from simple stop smoking and weight reduction problems to severe phobic and anxiety cases. When used with skill, ego state therapy can provide approaches for handling borderline conditions in ways well beyond the scope of other therapies currently available or, for that matter, in any case where some measure of dissociation, mild or severe, is found.

REFERENCES

Adler, A. (1963). *The practice and theory of individual psychology.* Totowa, NJ: Littlefield, Adams.

Adler, G. (1948). *Studies in analytical psychology.* London, England: Routledge & Kegan Paul.

Alexander, F., & French, T. M. (1946). *Psychoanalytic therapy.* New York: Ronald Press.

Allison, R. B. (1974). A new treatment approach for multiple personalities. *American Journal of Clinical Hypnosis, 17,* 15–32.

American Psychiatric Association. (1994). *Diagnostic and statistical manual of mental disorders* (4th ed.). Washington, DC: Author.

American Psychiatric Association. (2000). *Diagnostic and statistical manual of mental disorders* (4th ed.) *text revision.* Washington, DC: Author.

Amundson, J. K., Aladin, A., & Gill, E. (2003). Efficacy vs. effectiveness research in psychotherapy: Implications for clinical hypnosis. *American Journal of Clinical Hypnosis. 46*(1), 11–31.

As, A. (1962). The recovery of forgotten language knowledge through hypnotic age regression. *American Journal of Clinical Hypnosis, 5,* 21–29.

Aston-Jones, G., Rajkowski, R., & Cohen, J. (1999). Role of locus coeruleus in attention and behavioral flexibility. *Biological Psychiatry, 46,* 1309–1320.

Baker, E. L. (1981). A hypnotherapeutic approach to enhance object relatedness in psychotic patients. *International Journal of Clinical and Experimental Hypnosis, 29,* 136–147.

Baker, E. L. (1983a). Resistance in hypnotherapy of primitive states: Its meaning and management. *International Journal of Clinical and Experimental Hypnosis, 31, 2,* 82–89.

Baker, E. L. (1983b). The use of hypnotic dreaming in the treatment of the borderline patient: Some thoughts on resistance and transitional phenomena. *International Journal of Clinical and Experimental Hypnosis, 31, 1,* 19–27.

Baker, E. L. (1983c). The use of hypnotic techniques with psychotics. *American Journal of Clinical Hypnosis, 25,* 283–288.

Baker, E. L. (2004). Personal communication to AFB.

Bandura, A., & Walters, R. (1963). *Social learning and personality development.* New York: Holt, Rinehart, and Winston.

Banyai, E. I., & Hilgard, E. R. (1976). A comparison of active-alert hypnotic induction with traditional relaxation induction. *Journal of Abnormal Psychology, 85,* 218–224.

Barabasz, A. (1970a). Galvanic skin response and test anxiety among Negroes and Caucasians. *Child Study Journal, 1,* 33–36.

Barabasz, A. (1970b). Temporal orientation and academic achievement in college. *Journal of Social Psychology, 82,* 265–267.

Barabasz, A. (1970c). Time estimation in delinquents and non-delinquents. *Journal of General Psychology, 82,* 265–267.

Barabasz, A. (1974a). Enhancement of temporal orientation through exposure to audio tape recorded counseling models. *Adolescence, 9,* 107–112.

Barabasz, A. (1974b). Enlarging temporal orientation: A test of alternative counseling approaches. *Journal of Social Psychology, 93,* 67–64.

Barabasz, A. (1974c). Quantifying hierarchy stimuli in systematic desensitization via GSR: A preliminary investigation. *Child Study Journal, 4,* 201–211.

Barabasz, A. (1977). *New techniques in behavior therapy and hypnosis.* South Orange, NJ: Power Publishers.

Barabasz, A. (1979). Isolation, EEG alpha and hypnotizability in Antarctica. In Burrows, G., (Eds.) *Hypnosis 1979* (pp. 3–18), Amsterdam: Elsevier/North Holland Biomedical Press.

Barabasz, A. (1980a). Effects of hypnosis and perceptual deprivation on vigilance in a simulated radar target detection task. *Perceptual and Motor Skills, 50,* 19–24.

Barabasz, A. (1980b). EEG alpha, skin conductance and hypnotizability in Antarctica. *International Journal of Clinical and Experimental Hypnosis, 28,* 63–74.

Barabasz, A. (1980c). Enhancement of hypnotic susceptibility following perceptual deprivation: Pain tolerance, electrodermal and EEG correlates. In Pajntar, M., Roskar, E., Lavric, M., (Eds.) *Hypnosis in psychotherapy and psychosomatic medicine* (pp. 13–18). Ljubljana, Yugoslavia: University Press (Univerzitetna tiskarna).

Barabasz, A. (1980d). Imaginative involvement and hypnotizability in Antarctica. Proceedings—10th Annual Congress of the Australian Society for Clinical and Experimental Hypnosis, Hobart, Tasmania, September.

Barabasz, A. (1982). Restricted environmental stimulation and the enhancement of hypnotizability: Pain, EEG alpha, skin conductance and temperature responses. *International Journal of Clinical and Experimental Hypnosis, 30*(2), 147–166.

Barabasz, A. (1984a). Antarctic isolation and imaginative involvement: Preliminary findings. *International Journal of Clinical and Experimental Hypnosis, 32,* 296–300.

Barabasz, A. (1984b). Hypnosis in the Treatment of HPV. Presented at Massachusetts General Hospital, Boston, April 7.

Barabasz, A. (1994). Schnell neuronale Aktivierung. Reduzierte Stimulation und psychophysiologische Aufziechnungen bei der Behandlung eines phobischen Piloten. *Experimentelle und Klinische Hypnose, 10,* 167–176.

Barabasz, A. (2000). EEG markers of alert hypnosis: The induction makes a difference. *Sleep and Hypnosis, 2*(4), 164–169.

Barabasz, A. (2002). Personal communication, August 11, from Erika Fromm.

Barabasz, A. (2003a). Presidential address: Hypnosis for real-induction can make the difference. 111th annual convention of the American Psychological Association, Toronto, August 7–10.

Barabasz, A. (2003b). The reality of trance. Keynote address: presented at the annual conference of the Australian Society of Hypnosis, Gold Coast, Australia, September 10–16.

Barabasz, A. (in preparation). Dream interpretation using "specific radiality": An extension of Watkins's technique.

Barabasz, A. (2008a). Abreaction and age regression in hypnoanalysis and Ego State Therapy. Plenary Session Address. German Annual National Hypnosis Congress, Milton Erickson Foundation Jahrestagung der Milton-Erickson-Gesellschaft fuer Klinische Hypnose, March 6–9, Bad Orb, Germany.

Barabasz, A. (2008b). Invited Address: Ego-State Therapy and Hypnoanalysis. Presented at the 116th American Psychological Association Convention, Boston, Convention Center, Boston, MA, August 15–17.

Barabasz, A. (2008c). Keynote address: Ego-State Therapy: Evocation of Child-like Affective States for Trauma Resolution. 5th German-Nepal International Medical Conference, HauptKongress, Kathmandu, Nepal, May 4–10.

Barabasz, A., & Barabasz, M. (1989). Effects of restricted environmental stimulation: Enhancement of hypnotizability for experimental and chronic pain control. *International Journal of Clinical and Experimental Hypnosis, 37*(3), 217–231.

Barabasz, A., & Barabasz, M. (1992). Research design considerations. In E. Fromm & M. Nash (Eds.) *Contemporary hypnosis research* (pp. 173–200). New York: Guilford Press.

Barabasz, A., & Barabasz M. (Eds.) (1993). *Clinical and experimental restricted environmental stimulation: New developments and perspective.* New York: Springer-Verlag.

Barabasz, A., & Barabasz, M. (1994a). EEG responses to a reading comprehension task during active alert hypnosis and waking states. Paper presented at the 45th annual scientific meeting of the Society for Clinical and Experimental Hypnosis, San Francisco, California, October.

Barabasz, A., & Barabasz, M. (1994b). Effects of focused attention on EEG topography during a reading task. Symposium: Behavioral Medicine, Psychophysiology and Hypnosis, presented at the 102nd annual convention of the American Psychological Association (APA Division 30), Los Angeles, California, August 12–16.

Barabasz, A., & Barabasz, M. (1996). Neurotherapy and alert hypnosis in the treatment of attention deficit hyperactivity disorder. In S. Lynn, I. Kirsch, & J. Rhue (Eds.) *Clinical hypnosis casebook* (pp. 271–292). Washington, D.C.: American Psychological Association.

Barabasz, A., & Barabasz, M. (2006). Effects of tailored and manualized hypnotic inductions for complicated irritable bowel syndrome patients. *International Journal of Clinical and Experimental Hypnosis, 54,* 100–112.

Barabasz, A., Barabasz, M., Jensen, S., Calvin, S., Trevison, M., & Warner, D. (1999). Cortical event related potentials show the structure of hypnotic suggestions is crucial. *International Journal of Clinical and Experimental Hypnosis, 47*(1), 5–22.

Barabasz, A., Barabasz, M., Lin-Roark, I., Roark, J., Sanchez, O., & Christensen, C. (2003). Age regression produced focal point dependence: Experience makes a difference. Presented at 54th annual scientific program, Society for Clinical and Experimental Hypnosis, Chicago, November 12–16.

Barabasz, A., Barabasz, M., & Rickard, J. (in preparation). Hypnosis relieves phantom limb pain.

Barabasz, M. Barabasz, A. & Mullin, C.S. (1983). Effects of brief Antarctic isolation on absorption and hypnotic susceptibility: Preliminary results and recommendations. *International Journal of Clinical and Experimental Hypnosis, 31,* 235–238.

Barabasz, A. & Christensen, C. (2006). Age regression: Tailored vs. scripted inductions. *American Journal of Clinical Hypnosis, 48,* 4, 251–261.

Barabasz, A., Crawford, H., & Barabasz, M. (1993, October). EEG topographic map differences in attention deficit disordered and normal children: Moderating effects from focused active alert instructions during reading, math, and listening tasks. Paper presented at the 33rd annual meeting of the Society for Psychophysiological Research, Rottach-Egern, Germany.

Barabasz, A., & Dodd, J. M. (1978). Focal point location and inversion perception among New Zealand Maori and Pakeha children at two age levels. *Journal of Psychology, 99,* 19–22.

Barabasz, A., & Gregson, R. A. M. (1979). Antarctic wintering-over, suggestion and transient olfactory stimulation: EEG evoked potential and electrodermal responses. *Biological Psychology, 9,* 285–295.

Barabasz, A., Gregson, R. A. M., & Mullin, C. S. (1984). Questionable chronometry: Does Antarctic isolation produce cognitive slowing? *New Zealand Journal of Psychology, 13,* 71–78.

Barabasz, A., & Lonsdale, C. (1983). Effects of hypnosis on P300 olfactory evoked potential amplitudes. *Journal of Abnormal Psychology, 92,* 520–525.

Barabasz, A., & Watkins, J. G. (2005). *Hypnotherapeutic techniques.* New York: Brunner-Routledge.

Barabasz, M. (1996). Hypnosis, hypnotizability, and eating disorders. Presented at the 47th Annual Workshop and Scientific Program of the Society for Clinical and Experimental Hypnosis, Tampa, Florida.

Barber, T. X. (1962). Toward a theory of hypnotic behavior: The "hypnotically induced dream." *Journal of Nervous and Mental Disease, 135,* 206–221.

Barber, T. X. (1965). The effects of "hypnosis" on learning and recall: A methodological critique. *Journal of Clinical Psychology, 21,* 19–25.

Barrett, D. L. (1979). The hypnotic dream: Its relation to nocturnal dreams and waking fantasies. *Journal of Abnormal Psychology, 88(5),* 584–591.

Barrett, D. L. (1988a). Dreams of death. OMEGA: *The Journal of Death and Dying, 19,* 95–102.

Barrett, D. L. (1988b). Trance related pseudocyesis in a male. *International Journal of Clinical and Experimental Hypnosis, 36,* 256–261.

Barrett, D. L. (1991a). An empirical study of the relationship of lucidity and flying dreams. *Dreaming: Journal of the Association for the Study of Dreams, 1(2),* 129–133.

Barrett, D. L. (1991b). Through a glass darkly: The dead appear in dreams. OMEGA: *The Journal of Death and Dying, 24,* 97–108.

Barrett, D. L. (1992a). Fantasizers and dissociaters: An empirically based schema of two types of deep trance subjects. *Psychological Reports, 71,* 1011–1014.

Barrett, D. L. (1992b). Just how lucid are lucid dreams: An empirical study of their cognitive characteristics. *Dreaming: The Journal of the Association for the Study of Dreams, 2,* 221–228.

Barrett, D. L., & Loeffler, M. (1992). The effect of depression on the manifest content of the dreams of college students. *Psychological Reports, 70,* 403–406.

Barrett, D. (1993a). The "committee of sleep": A study of dream incubation for problem solving. *Dreaming, 3*(2), 1–7.

Barrett, D. (1993b). The "committee of sleep": A study of dream incubation for problem solving. *Dreaming: Journal of the Association for the Study of Dreams, 3,* 115–123.

Barrett, D. L. (1994). Dreams in dissociative disorders. *Dreaming: Journal of the Association for the Study of Dreams, 4*(3), 165–177.

Barrett, D. L. (1995a). The dream character as a prototype for the multiple personality "alter." *Dissociation, 8,* 61–68.

Barrett, D. (1995b). Using hypnosis to work with dreams. *Self & Society. 23,* 4, 25–30.

Barrett, D. L. (Ed.) (1996). *Trauma and dreams.* Cambridge, MA: Harvard University Press.

Barrett, D. (1998). *The pregnant man: And other cases from a hypnoanalyst's couch.* New York: New York Times Books/Random House.

Barrett, D. (2002). The "royal road" becomes a shrewd short cut: The use of dreams in focused treatment. *Journal of Cognitive Psychotherapy, 16,* 1.

Barrett, D. L. (2001). *The committee of sleep.* New York: Random House.

Baker, E. L. (1981). An hypnotherapeutic approach to enhance object relatedness in psychotic patients. *International Journal of Clinical and Experimental Hypnosis, 29,* 136–147.

Barnier, A. (2002). Posthypnotic amnesia for autobiographical episodes: A laboratory model for functional amnesia? *Psychological Science, 13*(3): 232–237.

Beahrs, J. (1986). *Multiple consciousness: Chapter five in limits of scientific psychiatry: Role of uncertainty in mental health.* New York: Brunner/Mazel.

Beck, A. (1976). *Cognitive therapy and the emotional disorders.* New York: International University Press.

Belagrove, M. (1992). Scripts and the structural analysis of dreams. *Dreaming, 2,* 23–38.

Berkeley, G. (1929). *Essay, principles, dialogues.* New York: Scribner.

Berkowitz, L. (1973). The case for bottling up rage. *Psychology Today, 2,* 24–31.

Biddle, W. E. (1967). *Hypnosis in the psychoses.* Springfield, IL: Thomas.

Bills, I. G. (1993). The use of hypnosis in the management of dental phobia. *Australian Journal of Clinical & Experimental Hypnosis, 21*(1), 13–18. Retrieved June 13, 2005, from PsycINFO (1840-Current) database.

Blanck, G., & Blanck, R. (1974). *Ego psychology: Theory and practice.* New York: Columbia University Press.

Bliss, E. L. (1986). *Multiple personality, allied disorders, and hypnosis.* New York: Oxford University Press.

Boor, M., & Coons, P. M. (1983). A comprehensive bibliography of literature pertaining to multiple personality. *Psychological Reports, 53,* 295–310.

Bower, G. H. (1981). Mood and memory. *American Psychologist, 36,* 129–148.

Bower, G. H., Monteiro, K. P., & Gilligan, S. G. (1978). Emotional mood as a context of learning and recall. *Journal of Verbal Learning and Verbal Behavior, 17,* 573–585.

Bowers, M. K. (1961). Theoretical considerations in the use of hypnosis in the treatment of schizophrenia. *International Journal of Clinical and Experimental Hypnosis, 9,* 39–46.

Brady, J., & Rosner, B. (1966). Rapid eye movements in hypnotically induced dreams. *Journal of Nervous and Mental Disease, 143,* 28–35.

Braffman, W., & Kirsch, I. (1999). Imaginative suggestibility and hypnotizability: An empirical analysis. *Journal of Personality and Social Psychology, 77,* 578–587.

Braun, B. G. (Ed.) (1984). *The psychiatric clinics of North America* (Vol. 7): *Symposium on multiple personality.* Philadelphia, PA: Saunders.

Braun, B. G. (Ed.) (1986). *Treatment of multiple personality disorder.* Washington, D.C.: American Psychiatric Association Press.

Brenman, M., & Gill, M. M. (1947). *Hypnotherapy.* New York: International Universities Press.

Brom, D., Kleber, R. J., & Defares, P. B. (1989). Brief psychotherapy for posttraumatic stress disorders, *Journal of Consulting and Clinical Psychology, 57*(5), 607–612.

Brown, W. (1920). The revival of emotional memories and its therapeutic value. *British Journal of Medical Psychology, 1,* 16–19.

Brown, D. P., & Fromm, E. (1986). *Hypnotherapy and hypnoanalysis.* Hillsdale, NJ: Lawrence Erlbaum.

Brown, D., & Fromm, E. (1987). *Hypnosis and behavioral medicine.* Hillsdale, NJ: Lawrence Erlbaum.

Brown, D., & Frischholtz, E., et al. (1999). Iatrogenic dissociative identity disorder-an evaluation of the scientific evidence. *Journal of Psychiatry and Law, 27,* 549–637.

Buber, M. (1970). *I and thou.* New York: Scribner.

Buck, J. N. (1948). The H-T-P technique: A qualitative and quantitative scoring manual. *Journal of Clinical Psychology,* Monograph Supplement No. 5.

Bugental, J. F. T. (1967). *The search for authenticity: An existential analytic approach to psychotherapy.* New York: Holt, Rinehart & Winston.

Burton, A. (1972). *Interpersonal psychotherapy.* Englewood Cliffs, NJ: Prentice Hall.

Callaway, C., Lydic, R., Baghdoyan, A., & Hobson, J. (1988). Pontogeniculoocipital waves: Spontaneous visual system activity during rapid eye movement sleep. *Cellular and Molecular Neurobiology, 2,* 105–149

Cardeña, E. (in press). Anomalous experiences and deep hypnosis. In Proceedings of the conference on developing perspectives on anomalous experience. Liverpool, U.K.

Cardeña, E., Maldonado, J., van der Hart, O., & Spiegel, D. (2000). Hypnosis. In E. B. Foa & T. M. Keane (Eds.) *Effective treatments for PTSD: Practice guidelines from the international society for traumatic stress studies* (pp. 247–279). New York: Guilford Press. Retrieved June 13, 2005, from PsycINFO (1840-Current) database.

Cardeña, E., Maldonado, J., Van der Hart, O., & Spiegel, D. (2000). Hypnosis. In E. Foa, T. Keane, & M. Friedman (Eds.) *Effective treatments for PTSD* (pp. 407–440). New York: Guilford.

Cauttella, J. R., & Bennett, A. K. (1981). Covert conditioning. In R. J. Corsini (Ed.) *Handbook of innovative psychotherapies*. New York: Wiley.

Chambless, D., & Hollan, S. (1998). Defining empirically supported therapies. *Journal of Consulting and Clinical Psychology, 66,* 7–18.

Cheek, D. B. (1962). Ideomotor questioning for investigation of subconscious "pain" and target organ vulnerability. *American Journal of Clinical Hypnosis, 5,* 30–41.

Cheek, D. B., & LeCron, L. M. (1968). *Clinical hypnotherapy.* New York: Grune & Stratton.

Christensen, C., Barabasz, A., & Barabasz, M. (2009). Effects of an affect bridge for age regression. *International Journal of Clinical and Experimental Hypnosis (57)* 402–418.

Chu, J. A., & Dill, D. L. (1990). Dissociative symptoms in relation to childhood physical and sexual abuse. *American Journal of Psychiatry, 147(7),* 887–892.

Chu, J. A., Frey, L. M., et al. (1999). Memories of childhood abuse: Dissociation, amnesia, and corroboration. *American Journal of Psychiatry, 156(5),* 749–755.

Comstock, C. (1986). *The therapeutic utilization of abreactive experiences in the treatment of multiple personality disorder.* Presented at the 3rd International Conference on Multiple Personalities and Dissociative States, Chicago, IL: September 20, 1986.

Conn, J. (1959). Cultural and clinical aspects of suggestion. *International Journal of Clinical and Experimental Hypnosis, 7,* 175–185.

Cooper, L., & London, P. (1971). The development of hypnotic susceptibility: A longitudinal (convergence) study. *Child Development, 42,* 487–503.

Cooper, L., & London, P. (1973). Reactivation of memory by hypnosis and suggestion. *International Journal of Clinical and Experimental Hypnosis, 21,* 312–323.

Copeland, D. R. (1986). The application of object relations theory to the hypnotherapy of developmental arrests: The borderline patient. *International Journal of Clinical and Experimental Hypnosis, 34,* 157–168.

Crawford, H. (1991). The hypnotizable brain. Presidential address. Annual meeting of the Society for Clinical and Experimental Hypnosis, New Orleans, November.

Crawford, H. J. (1982). Hypnotizability, day dreaming styles, imagery, vividness, and absorption: A multidimensional study. *Journal of Personality & Social Psychology, 42,* 915–926.

Degun-Mather, M. (2003). Ego-state therapy in the treatment of a complex eating disorder. *Contemporary Hypnosis, 20(3),* 165–173.

Dewey, J. (1916). *Democracy and education.* New York: Macmillan.

Dhanens, T., & Lundy, R. (1975). Hypnotic and waking suggestions and recall. *International Journal of Clinical and Experimental Hypnosis, 23,* 68–79.

Dollinger, S. (1985). Lighting – strike disaster among children. *British Journal of Medical Psychology, 58(4),* 375–383.

Dunn, K. K., & Barrett, D. L. (1988). Characteristics of nightmares: Subjects and their nightmares. *Psychiatric Journal of the University of Ottawa, 13,* 91–93.

Ellenberger, H. F. (1970). *The discovery of the unconscious.* New York: Basic Books.

Ellis, A. (1962). *Reason and emotion in psychotherapy.* New York: Lyle Stewart.

Ellis, A. (circa 1990). Personal communication to AFB.

Ellis, A., & Grieger, R. (1977). *Handbook of rational-emotive therapy.* New York: Springer.

Emmerson, G. (2000). Advanced Methods in Hypnotic Practice, Australian Society of Clinical Hypnosis workshop conducted at Northbrook House, East Malvern, Victoria, Australia.

Emmerson, G. (2003). *Ego state therapy.* Williston, VT: Crown.

Emmerson, G. (2006). *Advanced skills and interventions in therapeutic counseling.* Norwalk, CT: Crown House Publishing Ltd.

Emmerson, G. J. (2000). The resistance bridge technique: An ego state induction that locates the origin of the problem. *Australian Journal of Clinical Hypnotherapy & Hypnosis, 21*(2), 115–125. Retrieved June 13, 2005, from PsycINFO (1840-Current) database.

Emmerson, G., & Farmer, K. (1996). Ego state therapy and menstrual migraine. *Australian Journal of Clinical Hypnotherapy and Hypnosis, 17,* 17–14.

Erickson, M. (1939). An experimental investigation of the possible anti-social uses of hypnosis. *Psychiatry, 2,* 391–414.

Erickson, M. (1952). Deep hypnosis and its induction. In L.M. LeCron (Ed.), *Experimental hypnosis* (pp. 70–112). New York: Macmillan.

Erickson, M. (1968). Deep hypnosis and its induction. In L. M. LeCron (Ed.), *Experimental hypnosis* (pp. 70–112). New York: Citadel Press, 70–112.

Erickson, M. (1967). *Advanced techniques of hypnosis and therapy.* New York: Grune & Stratton.

Erickson, M., & Kubbie, L. (1941). The successful treatment of a case of acute hysterical depression by return under hypnosis to a critical phase of childhood. *Psychoanalytic Quarterly, 10,* 539–609.

Erikson, E. H. (1964). *Insight and responsibility.* New York: Norton.

Evans, F. J. (1979). Contextual forgetting: Posthypnotic source amnesia. *Journal of Abnormal Psychology, 88,* 556–563.

Federn, P. (1952a). *Ego psychology and the psychoses.* New York: Basic Books.

Federn, P. (1952b). Narcissism in the structure of the ego. (Read before the Tenth International Psychoanalytic Congress, September 1, 1927). In P. Federn & E. Weiss (Eds.) *Ego psychology and the psychoses* (pp. 38–59). New York: Basic Books.

Fenichel, O. (1941). *Problems of psychoanalytic technique.* Albany, NY: The Psychoanalytic Quarterly.

Fenichel, O. (1945). *The psychoanalytic theory of neurosis.* New York: Norton.

Ferenczi, S., & Rank, O. (1924). *The development of psychoanalysis.* New York: Nervous and Mental Disease Publishing.

Fisher, C. (1974). Subliminal and supraliminal stimulation before the dream. In R. L. Woods & H. G. Greenhouse (Eds.) *The new world of dreams* (pp. 377–388). New York: Macmillan.

Fligstein, D., Barabasz, A., Barabasz, M., Trevisan, M., & Warner, D. (1998). Effects of hypnosis on recall memory: Forced and non-forced conditions, *American Journal of Clinical Hypnosis, 40* (4), 297–305.

Frankl, V. (1963). *Man's search for meaning.* New York: Simon & Schuster.

Frederick, C. (1999a). *Who is the dreamer? The countertransference trance in ego state therapy.* Paper presented at the Annual Meeting of the American Society of Clinical Hypnosis, Philadelphia, PA.

Frederick, C. (1999b). *The intelligent fellow who points: Ego State Therapy for the treatment of chronic pain.* Paper presented at the Annual Meeting of the American Society of Clinical Hypnosis, Philadelphia, PA.

Frederick, C. (2003a, March 22). *You are always in my heart: Grief as a resource.* Paper presented at the First World Congress of Ego State Therapy, Bad Orb, Germany.

Frederick, C. (2003b). Editorial. *American Journal of Clinical Hypnosis, 46*(1), 1–2, 75–82.

Frederick, C. (2005). Selected topics in ego state therapy. *International Journal of Clinical and Experimental Hypnosis, 53*(4), 339–429.

Frederick, C., & McNeal, S. (1999). *Inner strengths: Contemporary psychotherapy and hypnosis for ego strengthening.* Mahwah, NJ: Erlbaum.

Frederick, C., & Phillips, M. (September 2004). Ego state therapy workshop. European Congress of Hypnosis. Gozo/Malta.

Freeman, R., Barabasz, A., Barabasz, M., & Warner, D. (2000). Hypnosis and distraction differ in their effects on cold press or pain and EEG. *American Journal of Clinical and Experimental Hypnosis, 43*(2), 137–148.

French, T. M., & Fromm, E. (1986). *Dream interpretation: A new approach.* New York: International University Press. (Originally Basic Books, 1964).

Freud, A. (1946). *The ego and the mechanisms of defense.* New York: International Universities Press.

Freud, S. (1920). *Beyond the pleasure principle. Standard Edition, 18,* 1–64.

Freud, S. (1924). Further recommendations in the technique of psycho-analysis: Observations on transference love. In *Collected papers* (Vol. 2) (pp. 377–391). London, England: Hogarth Press and the Institute of Psycho-analysis.

Freud, S. (1933). On narcissism: An introduction. In *Collected papers* (Vol. 4) (pp. 30–59). London, England: Hogarth Press and the Institute of Psycho-analysis.

Freud, S. (1935). *A general introduction to psycho-analysis.* New York: Liveright.

Freud, S. (1938). *A general introduction to psychoanalysis.* New York: Pocket.

Freud, S. (1953a). On the history of the psychoanalytic movement. In *Collected papers.* (Vol. 1, pp. 287–359). London, England: Hogarth Press and the Institute of Psycho-analysis.

Freud, S. (1953b). The interpretation of dreams. In J. Strachey (Ed. & Trans.). *The standard edition of the complete psychological works of Sigmund Freud* (Vol. 4–5). London, England: Hogarth Press.

Freud, S. (1953c). A case of paranoia (dementia paranoides). In *Collected papers* (Vol. 3, pp. 390–416). London, England: Hogarth Press and the Institute of Ps.ycho-analysis.

Freud, S. (1961). The dynamics of the transference. In J. Strachey (Ed. & Trans.). *The standard edition of the complete psychological works of Sigmund Freud.* (Vol. 12, pp. 97–208). London: Hogarth Press. (Original work published 1912).

Freud S., *Collected papers* (Vol. 1, pp. 24–41). London: Hogarth Press and the Institute of Psycho-Analysis.

Freud, S., & Breuer, J. (1951). On the psychical mechanism of hysterical phenomena. In Fromm, Erich. *The forgotten language*. New York: Rinehart.

Fromm, E. (1977). An ego psychological theory of altered state of consciousness. *International Journal of Clinical and Experimental Hypnosis, 25*, 372–387.

Fromm, Erich. (1973). *The anatomy of human destructiveness*. New York: Holt, Rinehart, and Winston.

Fromm, Erika. (1968). Transference and counter-transference in hypnoanalysis. *International Journal of Clinical and Experimental Hypnosis, 16*(2), 77–84.

Fromm, Erika, & Kahn, S. (1990). *Self-hypnosis: The Chicago paradigm*. New York: Guilford.

Fromm, E. (2001). Personal communication to AFB.

Fromm, E. (1992). An ego-psychological theory of hypnosis. In E. Fromm & M. Nash (Eds.) *Contemporary hypnosis research* (pp. 131–148). New York: Guilford.

Gabbard, G. (2000). An empirical evidence and psychotherapy: A growing scientific base. *American Journal of Psychiatry, 158*, 1–3.

Gabbard, G. (2005). *Psychodynamic psychiatry in clinical practice*. Arlington, VA: American Psychiatric Publishing.

Gainer, M. J. (1992). Hypnotherapy for reflex sympathetic dystrophy. *American Journal of Clinical Hypnosis, 34*, 227–32.

Gill, M. M., & Brenman, M., (1959). *Hypnosis and related states: Psychoanalytic studies in regression*. New York: International Universities Press.

Gill, M. M., & Menninger, K. (1947). Techniques of hypnoanalysis, a case report. In M. M. Gill & M. Brenman (Eds.), *Hypnotherapy: A survey of the literature* (pp. 151–174). New York: International Universities Press.

Ginandes, C. (in press). Six players on the inner stage: Using ego state therapy with the medically ill. *International Journal of Clinical and Experimental Hypnosis*.

Glover, E. (1955). *The techniques of psychoanalysis*. New York: International University Press.

Gordon, M. (1973). Suggestibility of chronic schizophrenic in normal males matched for age. *International Journal of Clinical and Experimental Hypnosis, 21*(4), 284–288.

Green, J., Barabasz, A., Barrett, D., & Montgomery, G. (2005). Forging ahead: The 2003 APA definition of hypnosis. *International Journal of Clinical and Experimental Hypnosis, 53*(3), 259–264.

Greenberg, J. (1964). *I never promised you a rose garden*. New York: Signet.

Greenberg, J. R., & Mitchell, S. A. (1983). *Object relations in psychoanalytic theory*. Cambridge, MA: Harvard University Press.

Grinker, R., & Spiegel, H. (1945a). *Men under stress*. Philadelphia, PA: Blakiston.

Grinker, R., & Spiegel, H. (1945b). *War neuroses*. Philadelphia, PA: Blakiston.

Grof, S. (1975). *Realms of the human unconscious: Observations from LSD research*. New York: Viking Press.

Grof, S. (1980). *LSD psychotherapy*. Pomona, CA: Hunter House.

Grof, S. (1985). *Beyond the brain: Birth, death and transcendence in psychotherapy*. Albany: State University of New York Press.

Grossman, L. (2003). Can Freud get his job back? *Time Magazine*, January 20.

Gruenewald, D. (1971). Transference and countertransference in hypnosis. *International Journal of Clinical and Experimental Hypnosis, 19*, 71–82.

Gruenewald, D., Fromm, E., & Oberlander, M. (1972). Hypnosis and adaptive regression: A ego-psychological inquiry. In E. Fromm and R. Shor (Eds.), *Hypnosis: Research developments and perspectives* (pp. 495–509). Chicago: Aldine-Atherton.

Gunnison, H. (2003). *Hypnocounseling: An eclectic bridge between Milton Erickson & Carl Rodgers*. Norwalk, CT: Crown House Publishing.

Gunnison, H. (2004). *Hypnocounseling*. Norwalk, CT: Crown House.

Guntrip, H. (1961). *Personality structure and human interaction: The developing synthesis of psychodynamic theory*. New York: International University Press.

Gutheil, E. A. (1970). *The handbook of dream analysis*. New York: Washington Square Press (Originally Liveright, 1951).

Hall, C. W. (1953). *The meaning of dreams*. New York: Harper & Bros.

Harper, R. (1959). *Psychoanalysis in psychotherapy*. Englewood Cliffs, NJ: Prentice Hall.

Hartmann, H. (1955). Notes on the theory of sublimation. In H. Hartmann, *Essays on ego psychology*. New York: International University Press.

Hartmann, H. (1958). *Ego psychology and the problem of adaptation*. (D. Rapaport, Trans.) New York: International Universities Press. (Original work published 1939).

Heaton, K., Hill, C., Petersen, D., Rochlen, A., & Zack, J. (1998). A comparison of therapist-facilitative self-guided dream interpretation session. *Journal of Counseling Psychology, 45*, 115–122.

Heidegger, M. (1949). *Existence and being*. Chicago: Henry Regnery.

Heisenberg, W. (1958). *Physics and philosophy*. New York: Harper.

Hilgard, E. (1965). *Hypnotic susceptibility*. New York: Harcourt, Brace, and World.

Hilgard, E. (1977). *Divided consciousness: Multiple controls in human thought and action*. New York: John Wiley.

Hilgard, E. (1979). *A saga of hypnosis: Two decades of the Stanford Laboratory of Hypnosis Research 1957–1979*. Unpublished manuscript, Stanford University.

Hilgard, E. (1986). *Divided consciousness: Multiple controls in human thought and action* (rev. ed.). New York: Wiley.

Hilgard, E. (1992). Dissociation and theories of hypnosis. In E. Fromm & N. Nash (Eds.), *Contemporary hypnosis research* (pp. 69–101). New York: Guilford Press.

Hilgard, E. R. (1962). Lawfulness within hypnotic phenomena. In G. H. Estabrooks (Ed.), *Hypnosis: Current problems* (pp. 1–29). New York: Harper & Row.

Hilgard, E. R. (1990). Personal communication to Arreed Barabasz.

Hilgard, E., & Loftus, E. (1979). Effective interrogation of the eyewitness. *International Journal of Clinical and Experimental Hypnosis, 27*, 342–357.

Hilgard, E., & Tart, C. (1966). Responsiveness to suggestions following waking and imagination instructions and following induction of hypnosis. *Journal of Abnormal Psychology, 7* (3), 196–208.

Hilgard, E. R., & Nowlis, D. (1972). Contents of hypnotic dreams and night dreams: An exercise in method. In E. Fromm & R. Shor (Eds.), *Hypnosis: Research, developments, and perspectives* (pp. 510–524). New York: Aldine.

Hilgard, J. (1974). Imaginative involvement: Some characteristics of the highly hypnotizable and non-hypnotizable. *International Journal of Clinical and Experimental Hypnosis, 22*, 138–156.

Hilgard, J. R. (1970). *Personality and Hypnosis: A Study of Imaginative Involvement.* Chicago, IL: University of Chicago Press.

Hilgard, J. R. (1979). Imaginative and sensory-effective involvements in everyday life and in hypnosis. In E. Fromm & R. Shor (Eds.), *Hypnosis: Developments, research, and new perspectives* (pp. 482–517). New York: Aldine.

Hill, C., Dimer, R., Sess, S., Hillyer, A., & Seemann, R. (1993). Are the effects of dream interpretation on session quality, insight, and emotions due to the dream itself, to projection, or to the interpretation process? *Dreaming, 3*(4).

Hill, C., Napayama, E., & Wonnell, T. (1998). Effects of description, association, or combined description/association in exploring dream images. *Dreaming, 8,* 1–10.

Hobson, J. (1989). *Sleep.* New York: Freeman & Company.

Hobson, J., Hoffman, S., Helfand, R., & Kostner, D. (1987). Dream design and activation-synthesis hypothesis. *Human Neurobiology, 6,* 157–164.

Hobson, J., & McCarley, R. (1977). Brain as a dream state generator: An activation-synthesis hypothesis of the dream process. *American Journal of Psychology, 134,* 1335–1368.

Hochberg, J. E. (1978). *Perception* (2nd ed.). Englewood Cliffs, NJ: Prentice Hall.

Horton, Crawford, Harrington, & Hunter-Downs. (2004). Increased anterior corpus callosum size associated positively with hypnotizability and the ability to control pain. *Brain, 127*(8), 1741–1747.

Hume, D. (1963). *The philosophy of David Hume.* New York: Modern Library.

Hunter, M. (2004). *Understanding dissociative disorders. A guide for family physicians and health care professionals.* Williston, VT: Crown House Publishing.

Huse, B. (1930). Does the hypnotic trance favor the recall of faint memories? *Journal of Experimental Psychology, 13,* 519–529.

Jacobsen, E. (1964). *The self and the object world.* New York: International University Press.

Janet, P. (1889). *L'automatisme psychologique.* Paris, France: Felix Alcan.

Janet, P. (1907). *The major symptoms of hysteria.* New York: Macmillan.

Janov, A. (1970). *Primal scream: A revolutionary cure for neurosis.* New York: Putnam.

Jiranek, D. (1993). Hypnosis in the treatment of repressed guilt. *Australian Journal of Clinical & Experimental Hypnosis, 21*(1), 61–74. Retrieved June 13, 2005, from PsycINFO (1840-Current) database.

Johnston, A. M. (1991). *Tex Johnston: Jet age test pilot.* Washington, D.C.: Smithsonian Institution Press.

Jourard, S. (1971). *The transparent self.* New York: Van Nostrand Reinhold.

Jung, C. G. (1916). *Psychology of the unconscious.* New York: Moffat, Yard.

Jung, C. G. (1958). *Memories, dreams, reflections.* In *Collected works XXVII* (pp. 115–117). New York: Pantheon.

Jung, C. G. (1966). Chapter II: The eros theory. In *Two essays on analytical psychology.* New York: Pantheon.

Jung, C. G. (1969). A review of the complex theory. In *Collected Works. Vol. 8. The Structure and Dynamics of the Psyche.* Princeton, NJ: Princeton University Press.

Kahn, D., & Hobson, J. (1993). Self-organization theory of dreaming. *Dreaming, 3*(3), 1993.

Kant, E. (1934). *Critique of pure reason.* New York: Dutton.

Keet, C. D. (1948). Two verbal techniques in a miniature counseling situation. *Psychological Monographs, 148*(62), 294.

Kernberg, O. F. (1972). Early ego integration and object relations. *Annals of the New York Academy of Sciences, 193*, 233–247.

Kernberg, O. (1975). *Borderline conditions and pathological narcissism.* New York: Jason Aronson.

Kernberg, O. F. (1976). *Object relations theory and clinical psychoanalysis.* New York: Jason Aronson.

Kierkegaard, S. (1954). *Fear and trembling and the sickness unto death.* Garden City, NY: Doubleday Anchor.

Kihlstrom, J. (1987). The cognitive unconscious. *Science, 237*, 1445–1452.

Kihlstrom, J., & Evans, F. (1979). *Functional disorders of memory.* Hillsdale, NJ: Erlbaum.

Kihlstrom, J., & Hoyt, I. (1990). Repression, dissociation, and hypnosis. In J. Singer (Ed.) *Repression and dissociation: Implications for personality theory, psychopathology and health* (pp. 181–208). Chicago, IL: Chicago University Press.

Kirsch, I. (1991). The social learning theory of hypnosis. In S. J. Lynn & J.W. Rhue (Eds.), *Theories of hypnosis: Current models and perspectives* (pp. 439–465). New York: Guilford Press.

Kirsch, I. (1996). Hypnotic enhancement of cognitive-behavioral weight loss treatments: Another meta-reanalysis. *Journal of Consulting and Clinical Psychology, 64*, 517–519.

Kirsch, I., & Council, J. (1989). Response expectancy as a determinate of hypnotic behavior. In N. P. Spanos & J. F. Chaves (Eds.), *Hypnosis: The cognitive-behavioral perspective* (pp. 360–379). Buffalo, NY: Prometheus Books.

Kirsch, I., & Lynn, S. (1998). Dissociation theories of hypnosis. *Psychological Bulletin, 123*(1), 100–115.

Kirsch, I., & Montgomery, G., et al. Hypnosis as an adjunct to cognitive-behavioral psychotherapy: A meta-analysis. *Journal of Consulting Clinical Psychology, 63*(2), 214–220.

Kleinhauz, M., Whorowitz, I., & Tobin, Y. (1977). The use of hypnosis in police investigation. *Journal of Forensic Science Society, 17*(2–3), 77–80.

Kline, M. (1958). *Freud and hypnosis.* New York: Julian Press and the Institute for Research in Hypnosis.

Kline, M. V. (1967). Imagery, affect and perception in hypnotherapy. In M. V. Kline (Ed.), *Psychodynamics and hypnosis: New contributions to the practice and theory of hypnotherapy* (pp. 41–70). Springfield, IL: Thomas.

Kline, M. V. (1968). Sensory hypnoanalysis. *International Journal of Clinical and Experimental Hypnosis, 16*, 85–100.

Kline, P. (1972). *Fact and fantasy in Freudian theory.* London, England: Methuen.

Kluft, R. (1985a). *Childhood Antecedents of Multiple Personality.* Washington, D.C.: American Psychiatric Press.

Kluft, R. (1985b). Dissociation as a response to extreme trauma. In R. P. Kluft (Ed.), *Childhood antecedents of multiple personality* (pp. 66–97). Washington, D.C.: American Psychiatric Press.

Kluft, R. (1985c). The natural history of multiple personality disorder. In R. P. Kluft (Ed.), *Childhood antecedents of multiple personality* (pp. 197–238). Washington, D.C.: American Psychiatric Press.

Kluft, R. P. (1986). Clinical corner. *International Society for the Study of Multiple Personality and Dissociation Newsletter, 4,* 4–5.

Kluft, R. P. (1987). On the use of hypnosis to find lost objects: A case report of a tandem hypnotic technique. *American Journal of Clinical Hypnosis, 29,* 242–248.

Kluft, R. P. (1988). On treating the older patient with multiple personality disorder: "Race against time" or "Make haste slowly." *American Journal of Clinical Hypnosis, 30,* 257–266.

Kluft, R. G. (in press). Dissociative identity disorder. *International Journal of Clinical and Experimental Hypnosis.*

Kluft, R. P., Frankel, F., Spiegel, D., & Orne, M. T. (1988). *Resolved: Multiple personality disorder is a true psychiatric disease entity.* (Tape cassette.) Mineola, NY: American Audio Association.

Kohut, H. (1971). *The analysis of the self.* New York: International University Press.

Kohut, H. (1977). *The restoration of the self.* New York: International University Press.

Kolb, L. C. (1988). Recovery of memory and repressed fantasy in combat-induced post-traumatic stress disorder of Vietnam veterans. In H. M. Pettinati (Ed.), *Hypnosis and memory* (pp. 265–274). New York: Guilford Press.

Konzag, T. A., Baandemer-Greulich, U., Bahrke, U., & Fikentscher, E. (2004). Psychotherapeutic relationship and outcome in psychotherapy of personality disorders. *Zeitzschrift fur Psychosomatische Medizin und Psychotherapies, [Journal of psychosomatic Medicine And Psychotherapy]* 50(4), 394–405.

Kosslyn, S., Thompson, W., Constantine-Ferrando, M., Alpert, N., & Spiegel, D. (2000). Hypnotic visual illusion alters color processing in the brain. *American Journal of Psychiatry, 157,* 1279–1284.

Kramer, E. (1971). *Art therapy with children.* New York: Schocken Books.

Kris, E. (1952). *The psychology of caricature: Psychoanalytic explorations of art* (p. 188). New York: International Universities Press.

Kris, E. (1956). The recovery of childhood memories in psychoanalysis. *The psychoanalytic study of the child* (pp. 54–88). New York: International University Press.

Kroger, W. S., & Fezler, W. D. (1976). *Hypnosis and behavior modification: Imagery and conditioning.* Philadelphia, PA: Lippincott.

Kubovy, M., & Pomerantz, J. R. (1981). *Perceptual organization.* Hillsdale, NJ: Erlbaum.

Lang, E., & Rosen, M. (2002). Cost analysis of adjunct hypnosis with sedation during outpatient interventional radiological procedures. *Radiology, 222*(2), 375–382.

Lavoie, G., & Sabourin, M. (1980). Hypnosis and schizophrenia: A review of experimental and clinical studies. In G. D. Burrows & L. Dennerstein (Eds.), *Handbook of hypnosis and psychosomatic medicine.* Amsterdam: Elsevier/North Holland Biomedical Press.

Lazar, B. S., & Dempster, C. R. (1984). Operator variables in successful hypnotherapy. *International Journal of Clinical and Experimental Hypnosis, 33,* 28–40.

Lazarus, A. A. (1994) How certain boundaries and ethics diminish therapeutic effectiveness. *Ethics & Behavior, 4*(3), 255–261.

Leonard, G. (1968). *Education and ecstasy*. New York: Delta.

Levick, M. (1981). Art therapy. In R. J. Corsini (Ed.), *Handbook of innovative psychotherapies*. New York: Wiley.

Levy, J. (1974). Psychobiological implications of bilateral asymmetry. In S. J. Diamond & J. G. Beaumont (Eds.), *Hemisphere function in the human brain*. New York: Wiley.

Locke, J. (1963). *The works of John Locke*. Aalen, Germany: Scientia Verlag.

Loftus, E. F. (1979). *Eyewitness testimony*. Cambridge, MA: Harvard University Press.

Lorentzen, S., Sexton, H. C., & Hoglend, P. (2004). Therapeutic alliance, cohesion and outcome in a long-term analytic group. A preliminary study. *Nordic Journal of Psychiatry, 58*(1), 33–40.

Lowen, A. (1975). *Bioenergetics*. New York: Coward.

Luborsky, L., McLelen, A., Diguer, L., Woody, G., & Seligman, M. (1997). The psychotherapists matters: Comparisons of outcomes across twenty-two therapists and seven patient samples. *Clinical Psychology: Research and Practice, 4,* 53–56.

Lynn, S. J., Kirsch, I., Barabasz, A., Cardena, E., & Patterson, D. (2000). Hypnosis as an empirically supported clinical intervention: The state of the evidence and a look to the future. *International Journal of Clinical and Experimental Hypnosis, 12,* 53–66.

Machover, K. (1948). *Personality projections in the drawing of the human figure*. Springfield, IL: Thomas.

Mahler, M. S. (1972). On the first three subphases of the separation-individuation process. *International Journal of Psychoanalysis, 53,* 333–338.

Mahoney, M. F. (1976). *The meaning in dreams and dreaming*. Secaucus, NJ: Citadel Press.

Malmo, C. (1990). Recovering the past: Using hypnosis to heal childhood trauma. In T. A. Laidlaw & C. Malmo (Eds.), *Healing voices: Feminist approaches to therapy with women. The Jossey-Bass social and behavioral science series* (pp. 194–220). San Francisco, CA: Jossey-Bass.

Malmo, C. (1991). Ego state therapy: A model for overcoming childhood trauma. *Hypnos, 28,* 39–44

Malon, D. W., & Berardi, D. (1987). Hypnosis with self-cutters. *American Journal of Psychotherapy, 41*(4), 531–541.

Mamelak, A., & Hobson, J. (1989). Nightcap: A home-based sleep monitoring system. *Sleep, 12,* 157–166.

Marcel, G. (1948). *The philosophy of existence*. London, England: Harvill.

Markowitz, J., & Street, L. (1999, October 15). NIMH propels psychotherapy research on a new courts. *Psychiatric News,* 20.

Mauron, A. (2001). Is the genome the secular equivalent of the soul? *Science, 291,* 831–832.

May, R. (Ed.) (1958). *Existence: A new dimension in psychiatry and psychology*. New York: Basic Books.

McKenzie, S. (1994). Hypnotherapy for vomiting phobia in a 40-year-old woman. *Contemporary Hypnosis, 11*(1), 37–40.

Means, J. R., et al. (1986). Dream interpretation. *Psychotherapy, 23,* 448–452.

Meares, A. (1957). *Hypnography: A study of the therapeutic use of hypnotic painting.* Springfield, IL: Thomas.

Meares, A. (1960). *Shapes of sanity.* Springfield, IL: Thomas.

Meares, A. (1976). *A system of medical hypnosis.* New York: Julian Press. (Originally Julian Press, 1961).

Meichenbaum, D. (1977). *Cognitive behavior modification: An integrative approach.* New York: Plenum.

Meissner, W. (1991). *What is effective in psychoanalytic therapy: The move from interpretation to relation.* North Vail, NJ: Jason Aronson.

Menninger, K., & Holzman, P. S. (1973). *Theory of psychoanalytic technique* (2nd ed.). New York: Basic Books.

Messerschmidt, R. (1927–1928). A quantitative investigation of the alleged independent operation of conscious and subconscious processes. *Journal of Abnormal and Social Psychology, 22,* 325–340.

Miller, M. C. (2004). Questions & answers. How important is the therapeutic alliance for the outcome of psychotherapy, and how should it affect a patient's choice of therapist? *Harvard Mental Health Letter, 21*(3, September), 7.

Miller, M., Barabasz, A., & Barabasz, M. (1991). Effects of active alert and relaxation hypnotic inductions on cold pressor pain. *American Psychological Association, 100,* 223–226.

Milne, G. (1985). Horse sense in psychotherapy. *Australian Journal of Clinical & Experimental Hypnosis, 13*(2), 132–134.

Moreno, J. L. (1946). *Psycho-drama.* New York: Random House.

Moreno, J. L., & Enneis, J. M. (1950). *Hypnodrama and psychodrama. Psychodrama Monographs, No. 27,* New York: Beacon House.

Morgan, A., & Hilgard, J. (1975). The Stanford Hypnotic Clinical Scale for Adults. In E. Hilgard & J. Hilgard (Eds.), *Hypnosis in the relief of pain* (pp. 134–147). Los Altos, CA: Kaufmann.

Moss, C. S. (1961). Experimental paradigms for the hypnotic investigation of dream symbolism. *International Journal of Clinical and Experimental Hypnosis, 9,* 105–117.

Moss, C. S. (1967). *The hypnotic investigation of dreams.* New York: Wiley.

Moss, C. S. (1970). *Dreams, images, and fantasy: A semantic differential casebook.* Chicago, IL: University of Illinois Press.

Mullin, C. S. (1960). Some psychological aspects of isolated Antarctic living. *American Journal of Psychiatry, 117,* 323–325.

Murray-Jobsis, J. (1984). Hypnosis with severely disturbed patients. In W. C. Wester & A. H. Smith (Eds.), *Clinical hypnosis: A multidisciplinary approach.* Philadelphia, PA: Lippincott.

Murray-Jobsis, J. (1988). Hypnosis as a function of adaptive regression and of transference: An integrated theoretical model. *American Journal of Clinical Hypnosis, 30,* 241–247.

Nash, M. (1987). What, if anything, is regressed about hypnotic age regression? A review of the empirical literature. *Psychological Bulletin, 102,* 1, 42–52.

Nash, M. (2005). The importance of being ernest when crafting definitions: Science and Scientism are not the same thing. *International Journal of Clinical and Experimental Hypnosis, 53,* 265–280.

Nash, M., Johnson, L., & Tipton, R. (1979). Hypnotic age regression and the occurrence of transitional object relationships. *Journal of Abnormal Psychology, 88,* 547–555.

Nash, M., Lynn, S., Stanley, S., Frauman, D., & Rhue, J. (1985). Hypnotic age regression and the importance of assessing interpersonally relevant affect. *International Journal of Clinical and Experimental Hypnosis, 33,* 224–235.

Naumberg, M. (1947). *Studies of the free art expression of behavior problem children and adolescents as a means of diagnosis and therapy.* New York: Nervous & Mental Disease Publishing Company.

Naumberg, M. (1950). *Schizophrenic art: Its meaning in psychotherapy.* New York: Grune & Stratton.

Naumberg, M. (1953). *Psychoneurotic art: Its function in psychotherapy.* New York: Grune & Stratton.

Nichols, M. P., & Zax, M. (1977). *Catharsis in psychotherapy.* New York: Gardner Press.

Nunberg, H. (1932). *Allgemeine Neuronsenlehre auf psychoanalytisher Grundlage* (Principles of Psychoanalysis). New York: International Universities Press.

Olsen, P. (1976). *Emotional flooding.* New York: Human Sciences Press.

Orne, M. (1951). The mechanisms of hypnotic age regression: An experimental study. *Journal of Abnormal and Social Psychology, 46,* 213–225.

Orne, M. (1959). The nature of hypnosis: Artifact and essence. *Journal of Abnormal and Social Psychology, 16,* 213–225.

Orne, M. (1979). The use and misuse of hypnosis in court. *International Journal of Clinical and Experimental Hypnosis, 27,* 311–341.

Orne, M. (1979). On the simulating subject as a quasi-control group in hypnosis research: What, why, and how. In E. Fromm & R. E. Shor (Eds.), *Hypnosis: Developments in research and new perspectives* (2nd ed., pp. 519–566). New York: Aldine.

Orne, M. (1990). Personal communication to AFB.

Orne, M. T., Dinges, D. F., & Orne, E. C. (1984). *The forensic use of hypnosis.* Washington D.C.: National Institute of Justice.

Orne, M., Whitehouse, W., Dinges, D., & Orne, E. (1988). Reconstructing memory through hypnosis: Forensic and clinical implications. In H. M. Pettinati (Ed.), *Hypnosis and memory* (pp. 21–63). New York: Guilford.

Oster, M. I. (2003). Efficacy or effectiveness: Which comes first, the cure or the treatment? *American Journal of Clinical Hypnosis, 46*(1), 10.

Palson, O. (2006). Standardized hypnosis treatment for irritable bowel syndrome: The North Carolina protocol. *International Journal of Clinical and Experimental Hypnosis, 54,* 51–64.

Perls, F. S. (1969). *Gestalt therapy verbatim.* Lafayette, CA: Real People Press.

Pettinati, H. M. (1982). Measuring hypnotizability in psychotic patients. *International Journal of Clinical and Experimental Hypnosis, 30,* 345–353.

Pettinati, H., Kogan, L., & Evans, F. (1990). Hypnotizability of psychiatric inpatients according to two different scales. *American Journal of Psychiatry, 147*(1), 69–75.

Phillips, M. (1994). Developing a positive "transference" in treating posthypnotic patients. Presented at the annual meeting of the American Society of Clinical Hypnosis, Philadelphia.

Phillips, M., & Frederick, C. (1995). *Healing the divided self: Clinical and Ericksonian hypnotherapy for post-traumatic and dissociative conditions*. New York: Norton.

Piccone, C., Hilgard, E., & Zimbardo, P. (1989). On the degree of stability of measured hypnotizability over a 25-year period. *Journal of Personality and Social Psychology, 56*, 289–206.

Pope, K. S., Sonne, J. L., & Holroyd, J. (1993). *Sexual feelings in psychotherapy: Explorations for therapists and therapists-in-training*. Washington, D.C.: American Psychological Association.

Prince, M. (1906). *The dissociation of a personality*. New York: Longmans-Green.

Putnam, F. W. (1989). *Diagnosis and treatment of multiple personality disorder*. New York: Guilford.

Rado, S. (1925) The economic principle in psychoanalytic technique. *International Journal of Psychoanalysis, 6*, 35–44.

Raginsky, B. (1961). The sensory use of plasticine in hypnoanalysis (sensory hypnoplasty). *International Journal of Clinical and Experimental Hypnosis, 9*, 233–247.

Raginsky, B. (1962). Sensory hypnoplasty with case illustrations. *International Journal of Clinical and Experimental Hypnosis, 10*, 205–219.

Raginsky, B. (1963a). Hypnosis in internal medicine and general practice. In J. M. Schneck (Ed.), *Hypnosis in modern medicine* (pp. 29–99). Springfield, IL: Thomas.

Raginsky, B. (1963b). Temporary cardiac arrest under hypnosis. In M. Kline (Ed.), *Clinical correlations of experimental hypnosis* (pp. 434–455). Springfield, IL: Thomas.

Raginsky, B. (1967). Rapid regression to the oral and anal levels through sensory hypnoplasty. *International Journal of Clinical and Experimental Hypnosis, 15*, 19–30.

Rainville, P., Duncan, G., Price, D., Carrier, B., & Bushnell, M. (1997). Pain affect encoded in human anterior cingulate but somatosensory cortex. *Science, 277*, 968–971.

Rainville, P., Hofbauer, R., Paus, T., Duncan, G., Bushnell, M., & Price, D. (1999). Cerebral mechanisms of hypnotic induction and suggestion. *Journal of Cognitive Neuroscience, 11*, 110–125.

Rainville, P., & Price, D. (2003). Hypnosis phenomenology and neurobiology of consciousness. *International Journal of Clinical and Experimental Hypnosis, 51*(2), 105–129.

Ramonth, S. (1985a). Dissociation and self-awareness in directed day-dreaming. *Scandinavian Journal of Psychology, 26*, 259–276.

Ramonth, S. (1985b). *Multilevel consciousness in meditation, hypnosis, and directed day-dreaming*. Uppsala, Sweden: University of UMEA.

Rank, O. (1932). *Art and artist, creative urge and personality development*. New York: Knopf.

Rank, O. (1952). *The trauma of birth*. New York: Brunner.

Ray, W., & De Pascalis, V. (2003). Temporal aspects of hypnotic processes. *International Journal of Clinical and Experimental Hypnosis, 51*(2), 147–165.

Regardie, F. (1950). Experimentally induced dreams as psychotherapeutic aids. *American Journal of Psychotherapy, 4*, 643–650.

Reich, W. (1949). *Character-analysis* (3rd ed.). New York: Orgone Institute Press.

Reik, T. (1933). New ways in psychoanalytic technique. *International Journal of Psychoanalysis, 14,* 321–334.

Reik, T. (1948). *Listening with the third ear.* New York: Farrar.

Reik, T. (1956). *The search within.* New York: Grove Press.

Reik, T. (1957). *Of love and lust.* New York: Farrar, Straus & Cudahy.

Renee (Pseudonym). (1951). *Autobiography of a schizophrenic girl* (with analytic interpretations by Marguerite Sechehaye). New York: Grune & Stratton.

Rogers, C. (1951). *Client-centered therapy.* Boston, MA: Houghton-Mifflin.

Rogers, C. (1961). *On becoming a person: A client's view of psychotherapy.* Boston, MA: Houghton-Mifflin.

Rolf, I. (1978). *Rolfing.* Santa Monica, CA: Dennis Landman.

Ronk, O. (1932). *Art and artist, creative urge and personality development.* New York: Knopf.

Ronk, O. (1952). *The trauma of birth.* New York: Brunner.

Rorschach, H. (1949). *Psychodiagnostics.* New York: Grune & Stratton.

Rose, S. (1976). Intense feeling therapy. In P. Olsen (Ed.), *Emotional flooding* (pp. 80–95). New York: Human Sciences Press.

Ross, C. A. (1989). *Multiple personality disorder: Diagnosis, clinical features, and treatment.* New York: Wiley.

Rossi, E. L. (1972). *Dreams and the growth of personality.* New York: Pergamon Press.

Rossi, E. L., & Cheek, D. B. (1988). *Mind-body therapy: Methods of ideodynamic healing in hypnosis.* New York: Norton.

Rycroft, C. S. (1979). *The innocence of dreams.* New York: Pantheon.

Sacerdote, P. (1967). *Induced dreams.* New York: Vantage Press.

Sanders, S. (1986). The perceptual alteration scale: A scale measuring dissociation. *American Journal of Clinical Hypnosis, 29,* 95–102.

Sanger, W. (1989). The role of acetylcholine in use-dependent plasticity of the visual cortex. In M. Steriade & D. Biesold (Eds.), *Brain cholinergic systems.* Oxford, England: Oxford University Press.

Sarbin, T. (2005). Reflections on some unresolved issues in hypnosis. *International Journal of Clinical and Experimental Hypnosis, 53*(2): 119–134.

Satir, V. (1967). *Conjoint family therapy.* Palo Alto, CA: Science & Behavior Books.

Scagnelli, J. (1974). A case of hypnotherapy with an acute schizophrenic. *American Journal of Clinical Hypnosis, 17,* 630–63.

Scagnelli, J. (1976). Hypnotherapy with schizophrenic and borderline patients: A summary of therapy with eight patients. *American Journal of Clinical Hypnosis, 19,* 33–38.

Scagnelli, J. (1977). Hypnotic dream therapy with a borderline schizophrenic: A case study. *American Journal of Clinical Hypnosis, 20,* 136–145.

Scagnelli, J. (1980). Hypnotherapy with psychotic and borderline patients: The use of trance by patient and therapist. *American Journal of Clinical Hypnosis, 22,* 164–169.

Scagnelli-Jobsis, (1976). Hypnotherapy with schizophrenic and borderline patients. *American Journal of Clinical Hypnosis, 19,* 33–38.

Scagnelli-Jobsis, J. (1982). Hypnosis with psychotic patients: A review of the literature and presentation of a theoretical framework. *American Journal of Clinical Hypnosis, 25*, 33–45.

Scagnelli-Jobsis, J. (1983). Hypnosis with psychotic patients: Response to Speigel. *American Journal of Clinical Hypnosis, 25*, 295–298.

Schafer, D. W. (1981). The recognition and hypnotherapy of patients with unrecognized altered states. *American Journal of Clinical Hypnosis, 23*(3), 176–183. Retrieved June 13, 2005, from PsycINFO (1840-Current) database.

Schiff, S., Bunney, W., & Freedman, D. (1961). The study of ocular movements in hypnotically induced dreams. *Journal of Nervous and Mental Disease, 133*, 59–67.

Schilder, P., & Kauders, O. (1956). *A textbook of hypnosis* (p. 96). New York: International Universities Press.

Schneck, J. M. (1965). *Principles and practice of hypnoanalysis*. Springfield, IL: Thomas.

Schneck, J. M. (1974). Observations on the hypnotic nightmare. *American Journal of Clinical Hypnosis, 16*, 240–245.

Schneidman, E. S. (1947). *Make a picture story test* (MAPS). New York: Psychological Corporation.

Schreiber, F. R. (1974). *Sybil*. New York: Warner Paperback Library.

Schwing, G. (1954). *A way to the soul of the mentally ill*. New York: International University Press.

Sechehaye, M. (1951). *Symbolic realization*. Monograph Series on Schizophrenia, No. 2., International University Press.

Sechehaye, M. (1956). *A new psychotherapy in schizophrenia*. New York: Grune & Stratton.

Seruda, B. (1997). *Empathic brief psychotherapy*. Northvale, NJ: Jason Aronson.

Shakow, D., & Rosenzweig, S. (1949). The use of the tautophone (verbal summator) as an auditory apperceptive test for the study of personality. *Character and Personality, 8*, 216–226.

Shapiro, F. (2001). *Eye movement desensitization and reprocessing: Basic principles, protocols and procedures*. New York: Guilford.

Shaw, H. L. (1978). Hypnosis and drama: A note on a novel use of self-hypnosis. *International Journal of Clinical and Experimental Hypnosis, 26*, 154–157.

Sherman, S. (1971). Very deep hypnosis: An experiential and electroencephalographic investigation. Unpublished doctoral dissertation. Stanford University.

Shevrin, H., & Luborsky, L. (1974). Subconscious stimulation before the dream. In R. L. Woods & H. B. Greenhouse (Eds.), *The new world of dreams* (pp. 371–377). New York: Macmillan.

Shor, R. (1979). A phenomenological method for the measurement of variables important to an understanding of the nature of hypnosis. In E. Fromm & R. Shor (Eds.), *Hypnosis: Developments in research and new perspectives*. New York: Aldine.

Shostrom, E. (1967). *Man the manipulator*. Nashville, TN: Abingdon Press.

Skinner, B. F. (1939). The verbal summator and a method for the study of latent speech. *Journal of Psychology, 34*, 33–38.

Smith, A. H. (1984). Sources of efficacy in the hypnotic relationship: An object relations approach. In W. C. Wester & A. H. Smith (Eds.), *Clinical hypnosis: A multidisciplinary approach* (pp. 85–114). Philadelphia, PA: Lippincott.

Smith, J., Barabasz, A., & Barabasz, M. (1996). A comparison of hypnosis and distraction in severely ill children undergoing painful medical procedures. *Journal of Counseling Psychology, 43*(2), 187–195.

Snyder, M. (1995). Self monitoring: Public appearances versus private realities. In G. Brannigan & M. Merrens (Eds.), *The social psychologist: Research adventures* (pp. 35–49). New York: McGraw-Hill.

Sonnier, I. (1982). Holistic education: Teaching in the affective domain. *Education, 103*, 11–14.

Spanos, N. P., & McPeake, J. D. (1975). Everyday imaginative activities on hypnotic susceptibility. *American Journal of Clinical Hypnosis, 17*, 245–252.

Sperry, R. W. (1973). Lateral specialization of cerebral function in the surgically separated hemispheres. In F. J. McGuigan & R. A. Schoonover (Eds.), *The psychophysiology of thinking* (pp. 209–229). New York: Academic Press.

Spiegel, D. (1981). Vietnam grief work using hypnosis. *American Journal of Clinical Hypnosis, 24*, 33–40.

Spiegel, D. (1983). Hypnosis with psychotic patients: Comment on Scagnelli-Jobsis. *American Journal of Clinical Hypnosis, 25*, 298–294.

Spiegel, D. (1984). Multiple personality as a post-traumatic stress disorder. *Psychiatric Clinics of North America, 7*(1), 1–110.

Spiegel, D. (1986a). Dissociating damage. *American Journal of Clinical Hypnosis, 29*(2), 123–131.

Spiegel, D. (1986b). Dissociation, double binds, and posttraumatic stress in multiple personality disorder. In B. Braun (Ed.), *Treatment of multiple personality disorder* (pp. 61–77). Washington, D.C.: American Psychiatric Press.

Spiegel, D. (1988a). Dissociation and hypnosis in post-traumatic stress disorder. *Journal of Trauma Stress, 1*(1), 17–33.

Spiegel, D. (1998b). Hypnosis and implicit memory: Automatic processing of explicit content. *American Journal of Clinical Hypnosis 40*(3), 231–240.

Spiegel, D. (2003). Negative and positive visual hypnotic hallucinations: Attending inside and out. *International Journal of Clinical and Experimental Hypnosis, 51*(2), 130–146.

Spiegel, D., & Barabasz, A. (1988). Effects of hypnotic hallucination on P300 evoked potential amplitudes: A reconciling conflicting findings. *American Journal of Clinical Hypnosis, 31*, 11–17.

Spiegel, D., Bierre, P., & Rootenberg, J. (1989). Hypnotic alteration of somatosensory perception. *American Journal of Psychiatry, 146*, 749–754.

Spiegel, D., & Cardena, E. (1991). Disintegrated experience: the dissociative disorders revisited. *Journal of Abnormal Psychology, 100*(3), 366–378.

Spiegel, D., & Classen, C. (2000). *Group therapy for cancer patients: A research-based handbook of psychosocial care.* New York: Basic Books.

Spiegel, D., Cutcomb, S., Ren, C., & Pribram, K. (1985). Hypnotic hallucinations alter evoked potentials. *Journal of Abnormal Psychology, 94*, 249–255.

Spiegel, H., & Shainess, N. (1963). Operational spectrum of psychotherapeutic process. *Archives of General Psychiatry, 9*, 477–488

Spiegel, H., & Spiegel, D. (2004). *Trance and treatment: Clinical uses of hypnosis* (2nd ed.). Arlington, VA: American Psychiatric Publishing.

Stampfl, T. G. (1967). Implosive therapy: The theory, the subhuman analog, the strategy, and the technique. Part I: the Theory. In S. G. Armitage (Ed.),

Behavior modification techniques in the treatment of emotional disorders. Battle Creek, MI: V.A. Publication.

Stava, L. (1984). The use of hypnotic uncovering techniques in the treatment of pedophilia. *International Journal of Clinical & Experimental Hypnosis, 32*(4), 350–355. Retrieved June 13, 2005, from PsycINFO (1840-Current) database.

Strachey, J. (1934). The nature of therapeutic action of psychoanalysis. *International Journal of Psycho-analysis, 15*, 127–159.

Strickgold, R., Pace-Schott, E., & Hobson, J. (1993). A new paradigm for dream research: Mentation reports following spontaneous arousal from REM and MREM sleep recorded in a home setting. Consciousness and Cognition, submitted.

Stekel, W. (1939a). *Sadism & masochism* (Vol. 1–2). New York: Liveright.

Stekel, W. (1939b). *Impotence in the male* (Vol. 1–2). New York: Liveright.

Stekel, W. (1940). *Sexual aberrations* (Vol. 1–2). New York: Liveright.

Stekel, W. (1943a). *Frigidity in women* (Vol. 1-2). New York: Liveright.

Stekel, W. (1943b). *Peculiarities of behavior* (Vol. 1-2). New York: Liveright.

Stekel, W. (1943c). *The interpretations of dreams* (Vol. 1-2). New York: Liveright.

Stekel, W. (1949). *Compulsion and doubt* (Vol. 1–2). New York: Liveright.

Stern, M. M. (1952). Art therapy. In G. Bychowski & J. L. Despert (Eds.), *Specialized techniques in psychotherapy.* New York: Grune & Stratton.

Stone, M. (1997). *Healing the mind: A history of psychology from antiquity to the present.* New York: Norton.

Suedfeld, P. (1980). *Restricted environmental stimulation.* New York: Wiley.

Sullivan, H. S. (1968). *The interpersonal theory of psychiatry.* New York: W. W. Norton.

Szechtman, H., Woody, E., Bowers, K., & Nahmias, C. (1998). Where the imaginal appears real: A positron emission tomography study of auditory hallucinations, *Proceedings of the National Academy of Sciences of the United States of America, 95*, 1956–1960.

Tart, C. T. (1964). A comparison of suggested dreams occurring in hypnosis and sleep. *International Journal of Clinical and Experimental Hypnosis, 12*, 263–289.

Tart, C. T. (1965). The hypnotic dream: Methodological problems and a review of the literature. *Psychological Bulletin, 63*, 87–99.

Teasdale, J. D., & Fogarty, F. J. (1979). Differential effects of induced mood on retrieval of pleasant and unpleasant events from episodic memory. *Journal of Abnormal Psychology, 88*, 248–257.

Tellegen, A., & Atkinson, G. (1974). Openness to absorbing and self-altering experiences ("absorption"), a trait related to hypnotic susceptibility. *Journal of Abnormal Psychology, 33*, 142–148.

Teyber, E. (2000). *Interpersonal process in psychotherapy.* Belmont, CA: Brooks/Cole.

Thigpen, C. H., & Cleckley, H. M. (1957). *Three faces of Eve.* New York: McGraw-Hill.

Tillich, P. (1952). *The courage to be.* New Haven, CT: Yale University Press.

Trussell, M. A. (1939). The diagnostic value of the verbal summator. *Journal of Abnormal Social Psychology, 34*, 533–538.

Tulring, E. (1983). *Elements of episodic memory.* Oxford, England, Clarendon Press.

Udolf, R. (1983). *Forensic hypnosis: Psychological and legal aspects..*Lexington, MA: D.C. Heath.

Ullman, M., & Zimmerman, N. (1979). *Working with dreams.* New York: Dela-corte/Eleanor Friede.

Vaillant, L. M. (1997). *Changing character: Short-term anxiety-regulating psychother-apy for restructuring defenses, affects, and attachment.* New York: Basic Books. Retrieved June 13, 2005.

Wadeson, H. (1980). *Art psychotherapy.* New York: Wiley.

Wadeson, H. (1982). Art therapy. In L. E. Abt & I. R. Stuart (Eds.), *The newer therapies: A source book.* New York: Van Nostrand Reinhold.

Walker, P. C. (1984). The hypnotic dream: A reconceptualization. *American Jour-nal of Clinical Hypnosis, 16,* 246–255.

Wark, D. M. (1998). Alert hypnosis: History and applications. In William J. Mat-thews and John H. Edgette (Eds.), *Creative thinking and research in brief therapy: Solutions, strategies, narratives, Volume 2* (pp. 287–306). Philadelphia, PA: Brunner/Mazel.

Watkins, H. (2001). Personal communication to AFB.

Watkins, H. H. (1978). Ego-state therapy. In J. G. Watkins (Ed.), *The therapeutic self.* New York: Human Sciences Press.

Watkins, H. H. (1980). The silent abreaction. *International Journal of Clinical and Experimental Hypnosis, 28,* 101–113.

Watkins, H. H. (2000). Clinical trials and follow-ups using the somatic bridge. Unpublished data. Missoula, MT.

Watkins, J. (1967a). Hypnosis and consciousness from the viewpoint of existential-ism. Chap. III in M. V. Kline (Ed.), *Psychodynamics and hypnosis* (pp. 15–31). Springfield, IL: Thomas.

Watkins, J. (1967b). Operant approaches to existential therapy. (Unpublished address.) Presented at the International Congress for Psychosomatic Medi-cine and Hypnosis, Kyoto, Japan, July 12.

Watkins, J. (1978a). Ego states and the problem of responsibility: A psychological analysis of Patricia W. *Journal of Psychiatry and Law,* 519–535

Watkins, J. (1978b). *The therapeutic self.* New York: Human Sciences Press.

Watkins, J. G. (1952) Projective hypnoanalysis. Chapter 19 in L. M. LeCron (Ed.), *Experimental hypnosis* (pp. 442–462). New York: Macmillan.

Watkins, J. G. (1971). The affect bridge: A hypnoanalytic technique. *International Journal of Clinical & Experimental Hypnosis, 19*(1), 21–27.

Watkins, J. G. (1992). *The Practice of Clinical Hypnosis, Volume II: Hypnoanalytic Techniques* New York: Irvington.

Watkins, J. G. (1995). Hypnotic abreactions in the recovery of traumatic memo-ries. *Newsletter of the International Society for the Study of Dissociation.*

Watkins, J. G. (1949). *Hypnotherapy of war neuroses.* New York: Ronald Press.

Watkins, J. G. (1954). Trance and transference. *Journal of Clinical and Experimental Hypnosis, 2,* 284–290.

Watkins, J. G. (1961). El puente afectivo: Una tecincia hipnoanalitica. *Acta Hyp-nologica Latino Americana, 2,* 323–329.

Watkins, J. G. (1963). Transference aspects of the hypnotic relationship. In M. V. Kline (Ed.), *Clinical correlations of experimental hypnosis.* Springfield, IL: Thomas.

Watkins, J. G. (1971). The affect bridge: A hypnoanalytic technique. *International Journal of Clinical and Experimental Hypnosis, 19,* 21–27.

Watkins, J. G. (1989). Hypnotichypermnesia and forensic hypnosis: A cross examination. *American Journal of Clinical Hypnosis, 32*, 71–83.

Watkins, J. G. (1992). Psychoanalyse, hypnoanalyse, ego-state therapie: Auf dur suche nach einier effektiven therapie. *Hypnose und Kognition, 9*, 85–97.

Watkins, J. G. (1995). Hypnotic abreactions in the recovery of traumatic memories. Newsletter of the International Society for the Study of Dissociation, *13*, 1, 6.

Watkins, J. (2005). *Emotional resonance. The story of world-acclaimed psychotherapist Helen Watkins.* Boulder, CO: Sentient Publications.

Watkins, J. G. & Barabasz, A. (2008). *Advanced hypnotherapy: Hypnodynamic techniques.* New York, London: Routledge.

Watkins, J. G., & Johnson, R. J. (1982). *We, the divided self.* New York: Irvington.

Watkins, J. G., & Watkins, H. H. (1978). *Abreactive technique.* (audiotape). New York: Psychotherapy Tape Library.

Watkins, J. G., & Watkins, H. H. (1979). The theory and practice of ego-state therapy. In H. Grayson (Ed.), *Short term approaches to psychotherapy* (pp. 176–220). New York: Human Sciences Press.

Watkins, J. G. & Watkins, H. H. (1980). *I. Ego states and hidden observers, II. Ego state therapy: The woman in black and the lady in white* (Audiotape and transcript). New York: Jeffrey Norton.

Watkins, J. G., & Watkins, H. H. (1981). Ego-state therapy. In R. J. Corsini (Ed.), *Handbook of innovative psychotherapies* (pp. 252–270). New York: Wiley.

Watkins, J. G., & Watkins, H. H. (1982). Ego-state therapy. In L. E. Abt & I. R. Stuart (Eds.), *The newer therapies: A source book* (pp. 137–155). New York: Van Nostrand Reinhold.

Watkins, J. G., & Watkins, H. H. (1984). Hazards to the therapist in treating multiple personality disorders. *Psychiatric Clinics of North America, 7*, 111–119.

Watkins, J. G., & Watkins, H. H. (1986). Hypnosis, multiple personality and ego states as altered states of consciousness. In B. W. Wolman & M. Ullman (Eds.), *Handbook of states of consciousness.* New York: Van Nostrand Reinhold.

Watkins, J. G., & Watkins, H. H. (1988). The management of malevolent ego states. *Dissociation, 1*, 67–72.

Watkins, J. G., & Watkins, H. (1997). *Ego states: Theory and therapy.* New York: Norton.

Watkins, J. G., & Watkins, H. (1998). Ego state transferences in the hypnoanalytic treatment of dissociative reactions. In M. Fass & D. Grong (Eds.), *Creative mastery in hypnosis and hypnoanalysis: A festschrift for Erika Fromm* (pp. 255–261). Hillsdale, NJ: Erlbaum.

Watkins, P. C., Matthews, A., Williamson, D. A., & Fuller, R. D. (1982). Mood congruent memory in depression: Emotional priming or elaboration. *Journal of Abnormal Psychology, 10*, 581–586.

Weiss, E. (1960). *The structure and dynamics of the human mind.* New York: Grune & Stratton.

Weitzenhoffer, A., & Hilgard, E. (1959). *Stanford Hypnotic Susceptibility Scale: Forms A & B.* Palo Alto, CA: Consulting Psychologists Press.

Weitzenhoffer, A., & Hilgard, E. (1962.) *Stanford Hypnotic Susceptibility Scale: Form C.* Palo Alto, CA: Consulting Psychologists Press.

Whalen, J. E. & Nash, M. (1996). Hypnosis and dissociation: Theoretical, empirical, and clinical perspectives. In L. K. Michelson & W. J. Ray (Eds.), *Handbook of dissociation: Theoretical, empirical, and clinical perspectives* (pp. 191–206). New York: Plenum.

Wilbur, C. B. (1988). Multiple personality disorder and transference. *Dissociation, 1,* 73–76.

Wilson, T. (1986). Effect of holistic and non-holistic teaching strategies on cerebral hemispheric laterality. (Unpublished dissertation). Washington State University.

Winncott, D. (1965). *The maturational processes and the facilitation environment.* New York: International University Press.

Wolberg, L. R. (1945). *Hypnoanalysis.* New York: Grune & Stratton.

Wolberg, L. R. (1948). *Medical hypnosis: Vol. I. Principles of hypnotherapy: Vol. II. Practice of hypnotherapy.* New York: Grune & Stratton.

Wolman, M. M. (Ed.) (1979). *Handbook of dreams: Research, theories and applications.* New York: Van Nostrand Reinhold.

Wolpe, J., & Lazarus, A. (1966). *Techniques of behavior therapy.* Oxford, England: Pergamon Press.

Woods, R. L., & Greenhouse, H. B. (1974). *The new world of dreams.* New York: Macmillan.

Woody, R. (1973). Clinical suggestion and systematic desensitization. *American Journal of Clinical Hypnosis, 15,* 250–257.

Wright, M. E. (with Beatrice A. Wright). (1987). *Clinical practice of hypnotherapy.* New York: Guilford Press.

Yalom, I. D. (1980). *Existential psychotherapy.* New York: Basic Books.

Zamore, N., & Barrett, D. L. (1989). Hypnotic susceptibility and dream characteristics. *Psychiatric Journal of the University of Ottawa, 14* (4), 572–574.

Zeig, J. (1974). Hypnotherapy techniques with psychotic in-patients. *American Journal of Clinical Hypnosis, 17,* 56–59.

Chapter 3

Hypnotic Dreams

Deirdre Barrett

Hypnosis and dreams have much in common, as is reflected in our language about them: "Hypnosis" is named for the god of sleep, phrases such as "dream-like" are scattered through hypnotic inductions and dream actions are sometimes described with words such as *trance*. Most references to non-pathological "hallucinations" refer to one or the other of these two states (Barrett, 1995). What they have in common is the coming together of the two major human modes of cognition:

1. The emotional, visual, irrational, hallucinatory, and intuitive mode of thought that Freud called "primary process," recently termed "right brain" thought in popular literature (with only the loosest relationship to actual hemispheric specialization).
2. Logical, verbal, linear reasoning that Freud called "secondary process," now popularized as "left brain thinking."

In deep hypnosis and lucid dreams (dreams in which the dreamer knows he or she is dreaming), these two processes are strongly manifested and integrated with each other. In deep hypnotic trance, the coexistence is achieved by starting in the logical waking state and introducing hallucinatory imagery; in a lucid dream it is achieved by starting in the primary process/hallucinatory mode and introducing secondary process logic. Although lighter hypnotic trances and normal dreams are characterized by more secondary process and more primary process respectively, they still involve a degree of coexistence of both modes not seen in most other states of consciousness—normal waking is mostly secondary process, psychosis is mostly primary process, and non-dreaming sleep shows very little of either. So hypnosis and dreaming already share much in common, but there is one area of interaction that is especially rich for these overlapping of modes of thought.

THE HYPNOTIC DREAM

A variety of hypnosis-related phenomena are sometimes referred to as "hypnotic dreams" including nighttime dreams influenced by posthypnotic suggestions and fantasies occurring spontaneously under hypnosis. This chapter will reserve the term for its most common usage—the result of an explicit direction to have a dream while in a hypnotic state. However, I'll return to some of these other potential relationships between dreaming and hypnosis in the last section.

The hypnotic dream was advocated as a therapy technique by many early psychodynamic hypnotherapists such as Milton Erickson, Jerome Schneck, Merton Gill, Margaret Brenman, and Erika Fromm. Erickson (1958) described a procedure he called "the rehearsal technique" in which he had a patient repeat over and over again a dream with the implied freedom of re-dreaming it in different ways. He believed that this served the dual purpose of progressively deepening the trance and of gaining insight into, and working through of, unconscious conflicts as the dream is reissued in less and less censored versions. For example, Erickson cites the case of a patient who had reported a dream in which he was in a pleasant meadow among comfortable warm hills. At the same time, the patient experienced a strong desire for something unknown and a paralyzing feat. On further elaborations, the locale changed to a valley with a little stream of water flowing under a horrible poisonous bush. Again the dreamer continued to look for something, while feeling terribly frightened, and getting smaller and smaller, as he was terrorized by the unknown that was pushing closer.

In the next repetition, the dreamer was a lumberjack picking up logs flowing down the river, and every time he obtained a log, it turned out to be just a skimpy little rotten stick compared to the big logs of other lumberjacks. In the next dream, he was fishing, and while everybody else caught big fish he only succeeded in obtaining a little sickly looking one that he was finally forced to keep.

Further repetitions eventually resulted in the disappearance of extensive amnesias and conscious blocking, and thus enabled the patient to reveal without further symbolism his inferiority feelings connected with stunted genital development and to discuss strong homosexual inclinations.

Sacerdote (1967a) describes a similar use of hypnotic dreams for rapid therapy, but stresses the experience of the dream as inherently therapeutic aside from any interpretation or insights gained from it. Some of his examples are very analytic and similar to Erickson's usage, while others involve an interpretation or breaking down of defenses. In the case of an obese elderly woman, she was told during the first and only hour of treatment under hypnosis: The dream will now start; you will be telling me all about that dream. In the dream you will see yourself having some very pleasant experiences, nice and slim as you want to be. What the dream will really be all about, it will be your own affair.

She reported the following dream: "I am in Paris, and then on the Riviera, and I am dancing and dancing; and then I went shopping, and ho! It is so wonderful; to get into clothes, size 10, and I had such a wonderful time." A second dream the same hour ran: "Oh, it is so wonderful, so wonderful; to be thin! Now I am on the beach and people are saying, 'What happened? Who are you? I don't recognize you.' I am just walking up and down on the beach and it is such fun; it is wonderful! Oh, I love the bathing suits!! I never could wear a bathing suit! Oh, that man! I do so want to go dancing tonight" (Sacerdote, 1967a, pp. 116–117). While the therapy was not quite limited to this one hypnotic session, it was after this one hour that she began to lose weight, becoming and remaining slim.

In a further article, Sacerdote (1972) reported the successful treatment of a long-standing case of insomnia that was apparently due to a fear of having nightmares by carefully inducing controlled dreams that let conflicts be expressed more gradually than in a full-blown nightmare.

Gill and Brenman (1959) described the use of hypnosis both for the production of original dreams and for the continuation of night dreams. In their technique the patients are told that they will continue a dream where it left off and that its meaning will become clearer. They gave the example of a young soldier discharged from the army in a state of depression and anxiety. He reported a dream of walking up a mountain path leading to a cave and trying to look inside, but waking up before he could see in. Under hypnosis, the patient looked in the cave and saw a witch who then becomes his mother, someone who was still somewhat frightening. Eventually, he was able to climb up on her lap and rest there like a young child. He then got up and walked away as a grown man. This dream was accompanied by great emotional expression and seemed to relieve his depression and anxiety greatly, the authors seeing the abreactive effect of the dream in this instance being the main component.

Berheim (1947) also stressed the abreactive effect of hypnotic dreams and offered an example in which he obtained good results by having a veteran go through a hypnotic dream about a real past traumatic memory of a battle and being wounded. He spoke out loud for himself and everyone else present as he reenacted the scene cathartically.

Lecron and Bordeaux (1947) described how hypnotic subjects could be instructed to dream on any specific topic. In a therapy setting, they believed that two of the most useful specifics were to have a person have a dream about their attitude toward a significant person or to have a dream about why resistance had appeared in an analysis. They report that an interpretable dream usually results from these suggestions that frequently speed up the progression of therapy.

Crasilneck and Hall (1975) reported helping a woman to find a lost locket by suggesting she would have a dream under hypnosis that would reveal its location. She had a dream in which she was looking at rows of books. Upon awakening, she remembered she had been reading a specific book the night the locket was lost, went to her bookcase, and found the locket marking her place.

Sacerdote (1968) described a group dream induction technique that he found helpful with patients who had trouble developing hypnotic dreams at first. He hypnotized a group and began with the people who easily produced dreams and they reported them out loud. He found that those who have had more difficulty dreaming can then, after hearing other dreams, begin their own dreams, which at the outset incorporate elements of the other patients' reports but go on to represent the dreamer's own unique material.

COMPARISONS OF HYPNOTIC AND NOCTURNAL DREAMS

These linear descriptions of the use of hypnotic dreams illustrate that it can be both an illuminating projective device for discovering conflicts and a helpful mode for working through these conflicts. How much the hypnotic dream resembles a more common therapy tool—the nocturnal dream—is a more difficult question.

An early review of the hypnotic dream literature (Tart, 1965) observed, at that time, that there was a lack of research concerning the equivalence or differences of hypnotic dreams from nocturnal dreams. Tart's review covered 34 publications in the area, only 10 of which he characterized as recognizing a need for some comparison of hypnotic dreams to nocturnal dreams. Of 14 studies drawing conclusions about this issue based on either anecdotal observation or theoretical assumptions, 10 asserted that hypnotic and nocturnal dreams are the same and 4 indicated differences.

It is quite clear that hypnosis is physiologically a waking state of consciousness rather than true sleep, although S. Kratochvil and H. MacDonald (1969) did find that posthypnotic suggestions could be carried out during sleep, suggesting that hypnosis can be superimposed with physiological sleep if explicit suggestions are given for this. Chapter 4 of this volume reviews neurological correlates of hypnosis in detail. However, there are several physiological findings specific to the hypnotic dream rather than characteristic of hypnosis in general. Two studies (Schiff, Bunney, & Freedman, 1961; Barrett, 1979) have reported that in highly hypnotizable subjects, hypnotic dreams are accompanied by movements that look indistinguishable from the Rapid Eye Movements (REMs) that accompany dreams during sleep. This raises the question of whether hypnotic dreams share any physiology with REM sleep. There is one physiological study comparing hypnotic dreams with other periods of hypnosis. De Pascalis (1993) reported Fast-Fourier spectral analyses of EEG readings from frontal, middle, and posterior electrodes placed on each side of subjects' scalps during hypnotic dream suggestions and during a resting trance state. With posterior scalp recordings, during hypnotic dreams, high hypnotizables displayed, as compared with the rest-hypnosis condition, a decrease in alpha 1 and alpha 2 amplitudes. This effect was absent for low hypnotizables. High hypnotizables during the hypnotic dream also displayed in the right hemisphere a greater 40-Hz EEG amplitude as compared with the left hemisphere; this effect was also absent in low susceptibles.

The majority of clinical writings on the use of hypnotic dreams are much more concerned with the degree of similarity of content and the psychological significance of hypnotic and nocturnal dreams than with their physiological correlates. Sacerdote (1968), the leading proponent of the use of the hypnotic dream stated: I have accepted on the basis of my experience that dreams hypnotically or post-hypnotically induced are psychodynamically equivalent and at times physiologically identical to natural dreams and therefore therapeutically valuable (p. 168).

Most of the clinicians dealing with this issue tended to agree on this equivalence; some state the assumption perfunctorily while others made elaborate arguments. Several theorists saw the equivalence as logically following from their theoretical concept of hypnosis. Fromm (1965) described their equivalence as resulting from both being primary process thought productions; she began her article "Dreams are 'the Royal Road to the Unconscious.' Freud was referring to ordinary nocturnal dreams but the same is true for the fantasies and dreams produced by hypnosis" (p 119).

Gill and Brenman (1959), while not arguing for an exact equivalence between hypnotic and nocturnal dreams, stated that since both hypnosis and dreaming are regressive states, this would facilitate switching easily from one to the other. They believed a person would be able to state unconscious conflicts more sharply via hypnotic dreams than in a waking state.

Schneck (1959) detailed his observations on the points of similarity between hypnotic and nocturnal dreams, stressing that all the same primary process mechanisms are employed:

> Hypnotic dreams may bear such close structural resemblance to nocturnal dreams as to be essentially indistinguishable from them. They may be simple or complex in concordance with the manner in which the patient tends to express himself in this fashion and in keeping often with the form and content of his spontaneous nocturnal dreams. The variety of dream mechanisms employed in the latter are evident in the former and the analysis of hypnotic dreams are often therapeutically beneficial. . . . Symbolizations, condensations, displacements and substitutions, representations by the opposite and a broader array of mechanisms are readily discernible. (pp. 156–157)

In another article, Schneck (1966) discussed the frequent arguement that hypnotic dreams are short, simple, and non-symbolic compared to the stereotype of intricate nocturnal dreamwork. He pointed out that in actuality, real nocturnal dreams also show this wide range of complexity. Schneck (1974) gave examples of the same individual's hypnotic nightmares (which occurred merely at the request for a dream under hypnosis) together with his nocturnal nightmares. Schneck concluded that both were structurally and dynamically equivalent, and that both dealt primarily with oedipal conflicts the patient was working through in an analysis with the author at that time. Both types of nightmares seemed to yield an equal number of associations and interpretations by the patient.

In two other studies, Schneck compared hypnotic dreams and nocturnal dreams with yet another category, the self-hypnotic dream, in which the subject would put himself into autohypnosis and suggest to himself that he would dream. Schneck found all three types of dreams were indistinguishable with respect to degree of activity, extent of embellishment, and nature of symbolizations. Furthermore, he found that all categories include sudden changes in locus, cast of actors, and types of action (Schneck, 1953). In another article, however, Schneck (1954) did allude to a difference he observed between hypnotic and self-hypnotic versus nocturnal dreams. He reported that in contrast to the nocturnal dreams, the two types of hypnotic dreams for one specific patient typically included lengthy conversational situations during which the patient spoke for herself or projected onto other various characters' different points of view about immediate problems.

Sweetland and Quay (1952) found that initial attempts at hypnotic dreams sometimes differed from nocturnal dreams but that after some practice, all subjects were able to produce dreams that they, the subjects, could not distinguish in any way from their night dreams. Mazer (1951) experimented with 26 subjects, giving them suggestions to dream while in hypnosis that specified that the dream would be "symbolic, with a disguised meaning." He concluded that while all hypnotic dreams were not exact duplications of nocturnal dreams, differences were minimal.

Mazer gave examples not only of the hypnotic dream but also of extensive associations and interpretations by the patients. He also reported a relationship between depth of the hypnotic trance and dream quality, finding that the more deep hypnotized the subject, the more symbolic and the more exactly like night dream was the hypnotic dream.

Domhoff (1964) reviewed studies near the same time as Tart (1964) pointed out that all empirical studies up to that time had looked only at hypnotic dreams, making unsupported assumptions about nocturnal dream content. He argued that not all nighttime dream content fit the stereotype. Domhoff suggested that hypnotic dreams likely differ no more from that stereotype than a representative group of nocturnal dreams from the same subjects might, and that the two categories could be equivalent.

Shortly after that, Moss (1967) conducted a survey that shows a narrow majority of diplomates in Clinical and Experimental Hypnosis (created by the American Board of Examiners in Psychology) equated hypnotic and nocturnal dreams. He received 46 replies from 52 diplomates canvassed in response to the question of whether they viewed hypnotic dreams as "similar in essential respects to nocturnal dream." The disagreement and uncertainty of these experts on the question is illustrated in the following distribution of his answers despite the majority agreement:

Some authors did propose specific differences between hypnotic and nocturnal dreams on theoretical grounds. Kanzer (1953), on a theoretical basis, argued that the setting of the hypnotic dream is bound to make it different from a spontaneous night dream. He stated: "On such induced dreams, the voice of the hypnotist takes the place of the day's residues, his ideas shape the latent thoughts, his comments give rise to the dream wish" (p. 231). Kanzer observed that dreams induced under hypnosis showed greater censorship than did spontaneous dreams. He also found that the form and imagery of the hypnotic dream were more typical of preconscious than unconscious mental activity.

Brenman (1949) also assumed that the context of hypnosis must have a significant effect on the dream. She stated: "In spite of the many similarities to night dreams in the formal structure of the hypnotic dreams, it must not be forgotten that while the primary function of the night dream is to guard sleep, the motive power for the hypnotic dream derives from the need to comply, in so far as possible, with the expressed wishes of the hypnotist; thus to guard an interpersonal relationship" (p. 458).

She belittled the assumption that hypnotic instructions to dream will result in a "real" dream, saying this employed the same logic as assuming that a hypnotic instruction to fly will result in real flight. She examined responses to the suggestion "You will now have a dream" and observed: "By and large, these productions employ 'primary processes' more than does normal conscious, waking thought but less than does the 'typical' night dream described by Freud. It might be said that often the hypnotic dream is a kind of second-rate poetry compared to this tight, complex outcome of the dreamwork. Thus, although a wide range of phenomena appears, it may be said, for the point of view of the formal qualities, that the average hypnotic dream takes a position which is intermediate between the conscious waking day-dream and the night dream" (p. 457).

Barber (1962) and Walker (1974) took a more extreme position—that the hypnotic dream is exactly the equivalent of a conscious waking day-dream. Barber asserted: the "hypnotic dream: is typically an unembellished imaginative product containing very little evidence of 'dreamwork.' In some instances it consists of straightforward previous happenings or of former night dreams; in the majority of instances, it consists of banal verbal or marginal associations to the suggested dream topic" (p. 218).

While Baber admitted he had occasionally seen hypnotic dream accounts that appeared to resemble nocturnal dreams, he offered the following three explanations for this resemblance:

1. They came from sophisticated subjects having great familiarity with Freudian dream theory who were likely to apply this to conscious productions.
2. Hypnotic dreams published in the literature were a few atypical ones selected from a large sample of failures.
3. The experimenters either implicitly, or explicitly, have given the expectation that they want their subjects to come up with elaborate symbolization.

Barber concluded by saying: "even with dreams suggested to deeply hypnotized subjects, it is difficult if not impossible to differentiate these from the imaginative productions of non-hypnotized controls who are instructed to imagine scenes vividly or to make up dreamlike material" (p. 219).

Walker (1974) wrote: "A more useful way of conceptualizing the hypnotic dream may be to see it as qualitatively no different from the response a person gives when simply asked to have a fantasy. . . . It is time that the knowledge about the hypnotic dream be integrated into the broader area of fantasy." Walker did not believe the hypnotic dream can be appropriately used in therapy in the manner a night dream would be interpreted. Instead, she suggests it be employed more in the manner of Desoille's (1965) "Directed Daydreaming," that is, as a kind of guided fantasy with systematic relaxation.

Tart (1964) found a difference in how easily nocturnal and hypnotic dreams could be influenced by topic. He had good hypnotic subjects listen to a tape-recorded narrative and told them to dream about it upon falling asleep that night and to have a dream about it immediately under hypnosis. Hypnotic dreams were found to conform much more closely to the narrative, although sleep dreams were also influenced.

Several researchers enumerated different types of "hypnotic dreams" of which only one type resembled the night dream. Tart (1966) and Gill and Brenman (1959) both suggested four such divisions. Tart categorized responses to suggestions as: (1) simply thinking about something, (2) daydreaming, (3) vivid hallucinations like watching a film, and (4) feeling "bodily located in a dream world."

He gave dream suggestions to both waking subjects and to those who had been through a hypnotic induction routine and then had them rate their own dreams as falling into one of these categories. A minority of subjects rated their experiences as feeling bodily located in a dream world even with hypnotic induction.

There was also a positive correlation of dream vividness to depth of hypnosis as measured by response to other hypnotic suggestions. However, there was no correlation between dream vividness and having gone through the induction routine. Tart criticized other studies on hypnotic dreams for defining hypnosis as having gone through hypnotic induction procedures; he believed it was more rightfully judged by the subject's state of consciousness.

Gil and Brenman (1959) distinguished four different types of productions issuing from the hypnotic instruction to dream. They were:

1. The embellished reminiscence.
2. The static pictorial image.
3. The quasi-allegory (which they described as resembling a conscious daydream but including in a rather obvious and primitive fashion some elements of unconscious symbolism).
4. The quasi-dream (which they said taken out of context is often indistinguishable from a night dream).

They found that analyzing all categories of productions was helpful in therapy, but did not conclude that even the fourth category is the exact psychodynamic equivalent of a night dream.

Spanos and Ham (1975) studied the characteristics of hypnotic dreams, working largely from a Barber-style theoretical orientation. They used 49 female student nurses at Medfield State Hospital (where Barber taught) as their subjects. All subjects were administered the Barber Suggestibility Scale (Barber, 1969) in a group setting. Their hypnotic dream reports, one per subject, were transcriptions of their verbal responses in an individual hypnotic session.

Following the "dream" session, all subjects rated the extent to which they (1) became involved in their imaginings, and (2) experienced their imaginings as an involuntary process. Furthermore, two judges independently rated the transcribed "dream" protocol of each subject for imaginative involvement. Judges also rated the "dream" protocols of 30 subjects for implausibility, fearfulness, and fragmentation. (The remaining 19 subjects had reported that nothing happened in response to the suggestion to "dream.") Subjects' self-ratings of "dream" protocols for involvement correlated highly with one another. Both involvement measures also correlated with self-ratings of involuntariness of imaginings and with Barber Suggestibility Scale scores.

The main emphasis, however, was upon how little dreamlike quality was involved in the hypnotic dream reports. Nineteen subjects experienced nothing, and of the remaining 30, the authors noted that: "for the overwhelming majority of these subjects a 'hypnotic dream' consisted of a plausible, non-fragmented, non-fearful, imaginary story" (Spanos and Ham, 1975, p. 47). The authors did mention that a few subjects reported "imaginings" that were implausible, fearful, and/or fragmented—another experimenter might have said more like nocturnal dreams, although they did not put it in those terms.

Spanos and Ham concluded by stressing a significant point: the often overlooked vast individual differences in response to the same instruction to "dream." They also concluded that hypnotic dreams were much like waking thought processes, without taking into account the brevity of the induction and instruction procedures or the biases of the people involved. The experimenters, and quite possibly the nurse-subjects, were already firm believers in Barber's idea that hypnotic phenomena should not viewed as something different from waking consciousness—the opposite bias of most researchers in other studies.

The one study that did in some way compare hypnotic and night dreams empirically was one by Hilgard and Nowlis (1972), however, they used different groups of subjects for the two categories of report. They collected hypnotic dreams in the course of administering the Stanford Hypnotic Susceptibility Scale, Form C (Weitzenhoffer and Hilgard, 1962). One step on this scale is an instruction to have a dream about the meaning of hypnosis specifically. Once the dreams were collected, Hilgard and Nowlis had subjects rate their own dreams on a three-point scale of vividness, counted the number of words in the dream accounts, and using Hall and Van de Castle's (1966) system, scored the number and categories of human characters in the dreams. They found 63 percent of their subjects rated their dreams as vivid as night dreams, 33 percent rated them like watching a movie, and 4 percent rated them like thinking or daydreaming. In order to compare these results to night dreams, Hilgard and Nowlis used the data of Hall and Van de Castle (1966) who had collected nocturnal dreams from a variety of subjects, including university undergraduates and prisoners. They were not well matched with Hilgard and Nowlis's subjects on age, geographic region, hypnotic susceptibility (on this potentially crucial variable, Hilgard and Nowlis's subjects were selected to score higher than the general population), or most other variables. The specification of the dream topic of the hypnotic dream only also negatively affected comparability. Hilgard and Nowlis acknowledged this as a rather unsatisfactory procedure, but characterized it as a pilot study that might indicate any gross differences among hypnotic and nocturnal dreams.

Hilgard and Nowlis did report several marked differences. Their hypnotic dreams were much shorter—a range of 13 to 238 words as compared to 50–300 for nocturnal dreams (though they failed to note that Hall and Van de Castle had tossed out dream reports under 50 words as too short to meaningfully score). The hypnotic dreams averaged 1.3 characters instead of the 2.6 Hall and Van de Castle reported for nocturnal, and the hypnotic dreams had fewer relatives as characters. The hypnotic dreams were also characterized by the authors as having more "Alice-in-Wonderland, psychedelic-type distortions." They did feel they were quite similar to nocturnal dreams in many ways and concluded that they are best considered as projective products falling somewhere between the Thematic Apperception Test (TAT) stories and night dreams.

A comparative study by Mixer (1961) reported no differences on "reality orientation" of deep trance subjects' hypnotic dreams versus night dreams. In his study, experienced clinicians independently rated the degree of reality orientation expressed in each dream as "impossible," "improbable," or "probable." Mixer interpreted the lack of significant differences in the two sets of data as indicating that "there is not difference in the degree of realism shown in hypnotic and nocturnal dreams of the same subjects, when their hypnotic dreams occur in a deep trance under conditions which duplicate night dreaming as closely as possible." Mixer did not use a medium trance group or draw any conclusions about whether hypnotic and nocturnal dreams would show the same reality orientation for them.

CONTENT OF HYPNOTIC, NOCTURNAL, AND DAY DREAMS FROM THE SAME SUBJECTS

This author undertook a study to explore how the content of hypnotic dreams, nocturnal dreams, and daydreams from the same subjects resembled or differed from one another and what depth of trance might play in this (Barrett, 1979). Sixteen university undergraduates, equally divided by both gender and capacity to achieve a medium versus deep trance by Davis and Husband (1931) criteria, were selected. No light trance group was included, as Hilgard (1965) has determined that a successful response to a suggestion to have a hypnotic dream falls near the beginning of the medium trance ranking. Subjects' ages ranged from 18 to 26 years.

During a six-week period, subjects were asked to write down the first three nocturnal dreams they remembered each week and their first three fantasies of daydreams in as much detail as they remembered. Once a week, the subjects were hypnotized and instructed three times during the session to have a hypnotic dream. After theses sessions, they were asked to write down everything they remembered of the hypnotic dreams. A few subjects failed to remember some of their dreams, so the total collected was 285 hypnotic dreams, 285 daydreams, and 277 nocturnal dreams.

All types of dream accounts were rated on scales from the Hall and Van de Castle rating system developed for nocturnal dreams. These included a three-point scale for setting—predominantly indoor, approximately equal, more of dream outdoors—and two-point scales for presence of certain types of characters—males, females, family, acquaintances, and strangers. Characters were recorded only for categories on which they were scorable.

For instance, "someone" appeared only in the total, not by gender and acquaintanceship categories. "A relative" would appear in the family category but not in the gender categories.

Other Hall and Van de Castle categories scored were two-point scales for hostility and friendliness on the part of other characters, and themes of anger, fright, sadness, happiness, or sexuality on the part of the dreamer. Reports could be scored as having none, any, or all of these characteristics present. For example, the following hypnotic dream report was rated by both raters as containing anger, fright, and sadness on the part of the subject: "I was in a boat alone on the lake. I was mad about something and was trying to drive away from it. I drove the boat until I saw an old man on the shore. I stopped and we went into his cottage and ate. We laughed until I was no longer mad. When I left it was dark. I couldn't see my way home so I stopped the boat. I looked straight up. The boat began to spin one way and I spun the other way. What little light there was closed in to a tiny circle and shot over to the left and disappeared" (Barrett, 1979a).

Other variables in addition to the Hall and Van de Castle system were used. Since the distinction of logic versus primary process thinking was often written about in the hypnotic dream literature, all categories of accounts were rated on a three-point scale of "distortion and illogical sequence" versus "coherence of story line." The following hypnotic dream was rated at the distortion end of the scale by both raters:

> I am standing on a beach or an island in the South Pacific. I turn around and notice that a group of people are chasing me. They chase me all over the island until I am trapped at the edge of a cliff which faces the ocean. I know that if I jump I will not be killed but still there is some fear of dying. Finally I jump off the cliff and into the water. Upon hitting the water I slowly float to the bottom of the ocean. When I get to the bottom I see a big orange fish which asks me what I am doing there. I tell the fish that I have come to learn. The fish then tells me that I am not ready and that I should go back. I then begin to float back up to the surface. [The dream ends.]

The following hypnotic dream was rated by both raters at the straight story line end:

> I was somewhere with my girlfriend and we were talking about her going away to that school. I was mentioning that I didn't want her to go away to that school. But I told her that I understood that she had to go where she'd be happy. And she turned all emotional and started crying and told me she was glad I was so understanding. And then she kissed me on the cheek and left to go inside. (My girlfriend was, in fact, up looking at this school the weekend I had the dream.)

Dream reports were rated on a three-point scale of activity versus passivity on the part of the dreamer. Passivity sometimes involved the dreamer being present in the dream but inactive, as in the following hypnotic dream scored "passive" by both raters: "I'm at a striptease show. The main 'attraction' comes out, and my friends and I cheer. She comes out dancing and wiggling about. Suddenly she pulled out a gun and began shooting people in the audience, yelling about 'male pigs' and getting revenge. We are all in a daze under chairs, but then she lays down her gun and finishes the dance."

Also rated as passive were dreams with the subject absent such at this nocturnal dream: "There were some horses running in a field. They were being led by a white stallion. This Stallion was very big and powerful. He kept running faster and faster. Until he began to fly. Then all of them were flying. They flew to the north till I couldn't see them."

As an example of a dream rated as very active by both raters was the following nighttime dream: "I'm lying in my bed—and hear sudden screams outside on the dimly little street. Being on the second floor, I jumped up and looked out and saw a woman being raped by a gorilla. Thinking I was awake, I ran outside and threw a paper cup at him and he fell over dead. I then jumped back up into my window and went back to bed."

The presence or absence of two other characteristics, unembellished memory and realistic planning, were rated on a two-point scale. An example of a report scored as unembellished memory by both raters was this hypnotic dream: "Images from a more recent event, spring break. Flying with my uncle in his Cessna Cardinal, four-seater aircraft. Vivid image of him, some feel of the place, interesting, exciting. Could look out the window and see the ground below clearly. Farms, wooden, white farm houses, roads, woods, ponds, fields, fences."

An example of a daydream report scored as realistic planning by both raters was: "The thought of getting a new stereo system has loomed across my mind quite often. Since I had never owned one, I was excited about getting one. It would be a Marantz or Pioneer cassette player-receiver. I seldom think of any other kind."

These ratings were done by two raters who did not know what type of dream a given report was. One rater did all 847 dream reports; the second rated one-third of the dream reports, equally distributed over subjects, style of dream, and week of experiment. Rater reliability was calculated for these 285 reports. High reliability was obtained, with rater agreement ranging from 92 to 100 percent for the different characteristics. The first rater's scores were then used for the statistical analyses. In addition, length in words was counted for all types of accounts by rater 1.

In two pre-experimental sessions, consistency of trance depth and rater agreement on visual observation of REM were checked. Subjects were found to be consistent in depth of trance reached, and raters agreed

100 percent on whether rapid eye movements were present for these 96 hypnotic dream periods (16 subjects × 2 sessions × 3 dreams). During the experimental period, the presence or absence of REM accompaniment during hypnotic dreams was noted by the experimenter only.

The ratings of each type of dream were averaged for every subject. Wilcoxon matched pairs signed ranks tests were done for all characteristics between the three types of dreams. In accordance with standard procedures for less than 25 pairs, Wilcoxon T scores were converted to Z scores for purposes of assessing statistical significance levels.

Table 3.1 presents mean ratings on each variable for the total group of subjects. Tables 3.2 and 3.3 report the mean ratings for deep and medium trance subjects, respectively. The categories of characters found in night dreams and hypnotic dreams were quite similar, and both differed from the characters found in daydreams. Table 3.4 presents Wilcoxon scores transformed to Z scores for these differences, which shows them to be significant. The greatest difference was that there were many more family members found in hypnotic and nocturnal dreams. There were also more strangers in them than in daydreams. There was a tendency for daydreams to average more acquaintances and fewer total characters, but neither of these trends achieved high statistical significance. In terms of the total number of dreams that had any characters, the only significant difference was that daydreams were slightly more likely to be totally without characters than were night dreams.

Emotional themes were similar between nocturnal and hypnotic dreams and different for daydreams (see Table 3.5). In the medium trance group, there were some differences between nocturnal and hypnotic dreams too. Hypnotic and nocturnal dreams got significantly higher ratings on anger, fright, and sadness—whereas daydreams were higher on happiness. Night dreams received somewhat higher ratings on fright and sadness than did hypnotic dreams. However, this trend on the total scores reflected only the medium trance subjects; the deep trance subjects' fear and sadness scores did not differ significantly between hypnotic and night dreams. There were no significant differences for the sexuality theme; it occurred about equally in hypnotic, night, and daydreams.

Attitudes of other characters showed similar trends to the subjects' emotions (see Table 3.6). Hostility of other characters was more common in nocturnal and hypnotic dreams than in daydreams. For medium trance subjects only, hostility was more common in nocturnal than in hypnotic dreams. Friendliness of other characters showed no significant differences among types of dreams.

The only significant difference in settings of dreams was that hypnotic dreams were more likely to be set outdoors than were nocturnal dreams. Distortion was much more common in hypnotic and nocturnal dreams than in daydreams (see Table 3.7). Action ratings were significantly higher for hypnotic and nocturnal dreams than for daydreams. For medium trance

TABLE 3.1 Means of Variable Ratings for Total Subjects

Variable	Dream Type		
	Hypnotic	Day	Night
Female family	.16	.04	.21
Male family	.22	.03	.13
Female acquaintances	.44	.43	.30
Male acquaintances	.54	.46	42
Female strangers	.39	.34	.50
Male strangers	.30	.23	.51
Distortion	1.49	1.07	1.48
Anger	.14	.04	.17
Fright	.24	.04	.38
Sadness	.10	.09	.23
Happiness	.41	.68	.26
Sexuality	.04	.12	.11
Hostility	.30	.13	.40
Friendliness	.36	.43	.30
Setting (1 = indoors, 3 = outdoors)	2.22	2.01	1.85
Any people present?	.69	.56	.78
Length in words	78.05	62.60	98.72
Unembellished memory	.21	.35	.12
Planning	.24	.49	.11
Activity = 1, Passivity = 3	1.72	1.51	2.20

subjects only, nocturnal dreams had a higher action rating than did hypnotic dreams. Planning and memory were both more common in daydreams than in nocturnal or hypnotic dreams. For the medium trance subjects only, they were both more common in hypnotic than in nocturnal dreams. Length in words for the total group was greater for hypnotic and nocturnal dream reports than for daydreams and greater for nocturnal than hypnotic dreams. There were not significant differences by gender in any of these trends.

REM was completely consistent for a given subject: it was observed as either 0 percent or 100 percent of their hypnotic dreams. All eight deep trance subjects and one medium trance subject exhibited REM accompaniment to dreams. The other seven medium trance subjects did not.

Thus, the clearest finding was the relation between depth of trance and the characteristics of hypnotic dreams. It is certainly possible that some characteristic not included in this study would show some differences between deep trance subjects' hypnotic and nocturnal dreams. However, it is clear the two categories have very much in common for this population. In psychotherapy, symbolic interpretation of deep subject's hypnotic dreams just as one would use on nighttime dreams is appropriate. Hypnotic dreams have the obvious advantages of ability to direct the topic of the dream and recall in patients who seldom remember nocturnal dreams. For medium trance

TABLE 3.2 Means of Variable Ratings for Deep Trance Subjects

Variable	Dream Type		
	Hypnotic	Day	Night
Female family	.17	.04	.24
Male family	.24	.03	.09
Female acquaintances	.44	.65	.27
Male acquaintances	.45	.58	.36
Female strangers	.28	.18	.64
Male strangers	.25	.12	.53
Distortion	1.56	1.04	1.49
Anger	.14	.01	.21
Fright	.32	.07	.36
Sadness	.11	.04	.27
Happiness	.32	.72	.22
Sexuality	.06	.04	.11
Hostility	.35	.16	.43
Friendliness	.37	.41	.31
Setting (1 = indoors, 3 = outdoors)	2.22	1.98	1.98
Any people present?	.68	.50	.71
Length in words	77.64	58.82	83.88
Unembellished memory	.17	.38	.12
Planning	.16	.46	.14
Activity = 1, Passivity = 3	2.15	1.63	2.16

subjects, the content differences between hypnotic and nocturnal dreams found in this study were great enough to indicate that hypnotic dreams cannot be used interchangeably in techniques designed for nocturnal dreams.

The distortion versus straight story line continuum in the present study bears a rough similarity to the psychoanalytic distinction between unconscious, primary process material versus conscious, secondary process thought. On the basis of the distortion scores, the medium trance hypnotic dreams can be viewed as having less primary process content than either nocturnal dreams or deep trance hypnotic dreams. The lower scores on negative themes of fright, sadness, and anger also support a conceptualization of the medium trance dreams as more closely aligned with normal waking consciousness than one's nocturnal dreams, although not as much as daydreams. These medium trance hypnotic dreams should not be used with the presumption that they are yielding predominantly unconscious material.

This awareness that hypnotic dreams are not really night dreams is implicit in many clinical hypnotic dream articles, though alternate suggestions, such as Walker's (1974) that hypnotic dreams be used more like guided fantasies are not completely appropriate either, as even the medium trance dreams still differ significantly in context from daydreams. The approach most indicated by the present study's findings on medium trance

TABLE 3.3 Means of Variable Ratings for Medium Trance Subjects

Variable	Dream Type		
	Hypnotic	Day	Night
Female family	.16	.03	.18
Male family	.21	.04	.18
Female acquaintances	.45	.22	.33
Male acquaintances	.63	.34	.49
Female strangers	.50	.49	.35
Male strangers	.34	.34	.48
Distortion	1.42	1.10	1.48
Anger	.13	.08	.13
Fright	.17	.02	.36
Sadness	.10	.14	.19
Happiness	.49	.66	.31
Sexuality	.02	.20	.10
Hostility	.25	.10	.40
Friendliness	.34	.42	.30
Setting (1 = indoors, 3 = outdoors)	2.22	2.04	1.72
Any people present?	.70	.63	.85
Length in words	78.46	66.36	113.55
Unembellished memory	.25	.32	.11
Planning	.32	.52	.08
Activity = 1, Passivity = 3	1.30	1.40	2.24

subjects would be to use their hypnotic dreams in a therapeutic medium designed specifically for them. In fact, this is what many clinicians seem to do. Approaches from Sacerdote's 1967a book onward advocate gaining insight from the projective qualities of hypnotic dreams in a manner that is not predicated on the basis of their being exactly like nocturnal dreams. This makes much use of the unique potential to request that the hypnotic dream be on a specific topic—which is possible with much more reliability than when using pre-sleep suggestions to influence nocturnal dreams. These techniques also use suggested repetitions and elaborations of hypnotic dreams that would not be possible with nighttime dreams. For medium trance subjects who do show major differences between night dream content and that in hypnotic trance, this type of technique would seem most useful. The one finding of my study that is inconsistent with the Hilgard and Nowlis (1972) study is in terms of comparing amounts of "distortion" between hypnotic and nocturnal dreams. I used a scale of distortion in terms of a break in logical sequence similar to the characteristics discussed as primary process. Hilgard and Nowlis had an "Alice-in-Wonderland, psychedelic distortion" scale that consisted largely of things changing size unexpectedly. I had assumed they would overlap, but on closer thought, this is not much like any characteristics of real nighttime dreams. It is

TABLE 3.4 Z Scores Between Average Frequencies of Types of Characters in Dream Reports

Type of character	Total Subjects	Deep trance Subjects	Medium trance Subjects
Total			
Hypnotic with day	−1.86	−.70	−.98
Day with night	−1.14	−.28	−1.12
Hypnotic with night	−.05	−.84	−1.18
Family			
Hypnotic with day	−3.18**	−2.37*	−2.20*
Day with night	−2.82**	−1.57	−2.20*
Hypnotic with night	−.71	−1.15	−.41
Acquaintances			
Hypnotic with day	−.11	−1.26	−2.03*
Day with night	−.62	−1.26	−1.26
Hypnotic with night	−1.66	−1.36	−.84
Strangers			
Hypnotic with day	−2.02*	−1.40	−1.40
Day with night	−2.43*	12.24*	−1.40
Hypnotic with night	−1.58	−1.54	−.07
Males			
Hypnotic with day	−1.81	−.70	−1.54
Day with night	−1.29	−.42	−1.54
Hypnotic with night	−.21	−.28	−.56
Females			
Hypnotic with day	−1.19	−.14	−1.12
Day with night	−1.34	−.70	−.98
Hypnotic with night	−.21	−.70	−1.12
Any characters present			
Hypnotic with day	−1.62	−1.44	−1.54
Day with night	−2.35*	−1.40	−2.03*
Hypnotic with night	−1.56	−1.12	−.56

* p<.05, two-tailed. ** p<.005, two-tailed.

more characteristic of films and hallucinogenic drug experiences. So it makes sense that there is more from the otherwise-less-like-nocturnal-dreams medium trance subject's hypnotic dreams. Since the deep trance dreams were so similar in all measured content to nocturnal dreams—including amount of irrational distortion and unpleasant affect intruding—it might seem reasonable to utilize more of the techniques developed for nocturnal dream while remaining aware that physiologically they're not from the same state.

A final note of interest in the content of the three categories of dream reports is that the group averages do not give any sense of the range of content; standard deviations offer a rough outline, but individual reports make clearer. As already discussed in this chapters, not all nighttime dreams fit the stereotype of distortion and primary process. But this was true for differences in daydreams. A few examples were extremely full of

TABLE 3.5 Z Scores Between Average Frequencies of Types of Emotional
Themes in Dream Reports

Emotional theme	Total Subjects	Deep trance Subjects	Medium trance Subjects
Anger			
Hypnotic with day	−3.06	−2.52*	−1.83
Day with night	−2.54	−2.37*	−1.18
Hypnotic with night	−.21	−.63	−.17
Fright			
Hypnotic with day	−3.41**	−2.52*	−2.37*
Day with night	−3.41**	−2.37*	−2.52*
Hypnotic with night	−3.08**	−.67	−2.37*
Sadness			
Hypnotic with day	−.97	−1.05	−.25
Day with night	−2.61*	−2.52*	−1.18
Hypnotic with night	−3.08**	−2.11*	−2.37*
Happiness			
Hypnotic with day	−2.02*	−2.52*	−1.12
Day with night	−2.43*	−2.52*	−2.52*
Hypnotic with night	−1.58	−.61	−1.86
Sexuality			
Hypnotic with day	−.92	−1.28	−1.78
Day with night	−.51	−1.46	−.84
Hypnotic with night	−1.84	−.91	−1.48

* $p < .05$, two-tailed. ** $p < .005$, two-tailed.

primary process—or other rare categories like fear and sadness. These differences are best illustrated with examples of the atypical dreams, so first, this is a nocturnal dream from one deep trance subject:

> Our fraternity was having a basketball game at Alumni Gym, and I was in the team. I was sitting on the end of the bench, and when one of our players was hurt, Steve decided to put me in. It took me awhile to get going, but finally I began moving pretty good. I wanted to score badly, so when I got the ball I shot and made it. The next time down court, I put a great move on my man and scored easily. Then when the opponent came down the court, and I dived after the ball, someone else dived after it too. He landed on my legs. His legs and mine became intertwined and he twisted my ankle. I had to be carried off the court.

In contrast to this narrative, which could pretty much describe a waking basketball game, the following daydream was reported by another deep trance subject—the first two sentences identifying type of account were stripped off for the raters but are printed here for relevance:

> This daydream occurred in Special Ed. Class. I wasn't actually asleep, but I was definitely in another world. I dreamed that I was in my

TABLE 3.6 Z Scores for Attitudes of Other Characters and Settings
of Dream Reports

Variable	Total Subjects	Deep trance Subjects	Medium trance Subjects
Hostile Characters			
Hypnotic with day	−3.01**	−2.03*	−2.52*
Day with night	−3.35**	−2.37*	−2.38*
Hypnotic with night	−1.36	−.00	−2.24*
Friendly Characters			
Hypnotic with day	−.83	−.56	−.70
Day with night	−1.29	−.91	−.98
Hypnotic with night	−.67	−1.79	−.17
Setting			
Hypnotic with day	−1.29	−1.12	−.84
Day with night	−1.29	−.28	−2.10*
Hypnotic with night	−3.01**	−1.52	−2.52*

* $p < .05$, two-tailed. ** $p < .005$, two-tailed.

house, upstairs, getting ready to go somewhere. My sister came to get me and bring me downstairs. I seemed to recognize the two visitors waiting downstairs. All I can remember is their big floppy hats covered most of their faces and their flowing dresses. I think that I was excited over their visit and I was about to go and greet them, but my instructor spoke to me.

REMs during hypnotic dreams also had a clear relationship to dream content. However, they corresponded so closely to whether the subject was from the medium or deep trance group that presence or absence of REM during hypnotic dreams was virtually synonymous with trance depth. Therefore, it's hardly a useful measure in research where experimenters are already assessing formal hypnotic depth by established scales. However, it may be very useful to observe REMs or lack thereof in clinical settings, where formal trance depth is rarely assessed, as this may indicate how deeply hypnotized the patient is and give a sense of how primary process the dream content is.

OTHER UTILIZATION OF HYPNOSIS WITH DREAMING

There are two other major ways in which hypnosis has been employed in combination with dreaming. The first—continuing or interpretation of a nocturnal dream in the hypnotic state—is much like the hypnotic dream. Hypnosis has been employed much like Jung's technique of "active imagination" to return to, continue, or elaborate on parts of a previous nocturnal dream. Hypnosis, as compared to doing these exercises in a usual

TABLE 3.7 Z Scores for Distortion, Action, Planning, Memory, and Length in Words of Dream Reports

Variable	Total Subjects	Deep trance Subjects	Medium trance Subjects
Distortion			
Hypnotic with day	−3.52**	−2.52*	−2.52*
Day with night	−3.41**	−2.36*	−2.52*
Hypnotic with night	−.27	−.83	−.67
Action			
Hypnotic with day	−1.98	−2.38*	−.21
Day with night	−3.52**	−2.52	−2.52*
Hypnotic with night	−2.67**	−.11	−2.52*
Planning			
Hypnotic with day	−3.30**	−2.52*	−2.20*
Day with night	−3.30*	−2.37*	−2.37*
Hypnotic with night	−1.73	−.21*	−2.20*
Memory			
Hypnotic with day	−2.56*	−2.52*	−1.18
Day with night	−3.30**	−2.52	−2.20*
Hypnotic with night	−2.17*	−.31	−2.37*
Length in words			
Hypnotic with day	−2.33*	−1.68	−1.68
Day with night	−3.52**	−2.52*	−2.52*
Hypnotic with night	−2.53*	−1.40	−2.24*

* $p < .05$, two-tailed. ** $p < .005$, two-tailed.

waking state, may heighten the experiential vividness of such experiences. With hypnosis, therapists sometimes give clients suggestions to reenter the dream and replay parts of it that are vague or forgotten. Some assume this is the actual nocturnal dream being recalled, but of course others suggest that new material might as easily be substituted. However, most agree that it provides interesting material for therapy whichever may be the case. One can also take a dream that seemed to terminate prematurely and suggest that it continue. This will result in an experience much like the "hypnotic dream" except that it begins with a topic determined by the dreaming mind the night before rather than by the waking ego of the dreamer or hypnotherapist.

Hypnosis can also be employed for even more direct interpretation of nocturnal dreams. Upon hypnotically "reentering" the dream scene, the dreamer can ask characters, "Who are you?" "What do you represent?" and "What are you trying to tell me?" They can look around a scene and ask: "What is this place" or "What real-life setting does this resemble?" Often quite unexpected yet crystal-clear answers come more directly than when pondering these questions from the more usual conscious "left-brain"/secondary process mode.

An example drawn from a woman in a brief workshop that I conducted illustrates some of these processes. Marge chose to work in this manner with a brief nightmare about her husband who had died six months previously. In the dream, Marge was in her house doing minor domestic tasks when the doorbell rang. She went to the door and opened it; there stood her dead husband. At this point she awakened in terror. Marge suffered both fright and intensification of grief for some time after this dream. Many bereaved people dream of lost loved ones, but usually these dreams are anywhere from bittersweet to deeply comforting to the dreamer (Barrett, 1991). The few frightening dreams about someone who has been much loved often contain some obvious element of the deceased beckoning the dreamer to join them in death. Marge's nightmare did not seem to have this element, and she did not immediately know what it was about the dream image or her feelings about her husband that had made it so terrifying.

In trance, I directed Marge to reenter the dream and instead of waking up at the crucial point, to ask the dream character who he was. Despite the obvious identification as her husband (characters usually give a rich array of answers that augment rather than replace the obvious identity), Marge's husband said, "I am joy." She was then instructed to ask what he had come to tell or show her and he said, "You can be joy, too." I then suggested she could interact with him or continue the dream in another way until it felt concluded. She proceeded to dance with him and then, bidding him goodbye, to go on dancing by herself before the dream ended.

Marge woke up smiling and began to relate a group of associations to the dream content to do with having always thought of her husband as the carefree, easy-going one in the marriage who knew how to enjoy himself and brought joy into her life. She realized that, in addition to the immense loss of him, she had been feeling that her own capacity to have fun had gone with him. She felt that the dream's image had given her the ability to have fun for herself in the future.

The other way in which hypnosis has been utilized in working with dreams is to use it to influence the content or recall of nocturnal dreams. Research by Charles Tart (1964) has found that hypnotic suggestions can influence future dream content. Hypnosis can be used to augment the same type of dream incubation procedures that are used without trance to shape dreaming toward solving a specific problem or for creative inspiration, however, the probability of achieving the desired content on a given night seems to be higher with hypnotic suggestion (Barrett, 1995). For example, a painter in one of my hypnosis and dream workshops found that with self-hypnotic suggestions to herself at bedtime, she could reliably produce dreams of paintings that she then replicated awake—phenomena that had occurred spontaneously but rarely for her previously.

Joe Dane (1985) demonstrated that hypnotic suggestions can increase the frequency of laboratory-verified lucid dreams. Zadra (1996) applied this to inducing lucidity to alter the content of recurring nightmares or help the dreamer wake from them.

I have found that it is easier to help someone alter recurring nightmare content toward other forms of mastery via hypnosis than it is to induce lucidity. With trauma patients who have nightmares that replay, at least partially, real events, rehearsal of changes in the dream during hypnosis can be very effective. In trance they practice a different ending to the dream in which they thwart a violent attack, tell off an abuser, remind themselves "this is not my fault" at some crucial moment, or say "this doesn't have to happen any more," and wake up. This hypnotic visualization, combined with the suggestion that at night the dream will happen much as it was "dreamed" in hypnosis, is often effective in altering even long-standing nightmares.

Many people have also utilized hypnotic and self-hypnotic suggestions for increased dream recall. Hypnotherapists often use this process with patients who begin as low dream recallers, using hypnosis both for direct verbal suggestions, such as, "You will find yourself remembering dreams easily and clearly when you wake up in the morning," and for imagery— picturing oneself finishing a dream, waking up with it clearly in mind as one reaches for a notebook, and watching oneself writing it down, and perhaps sketching images from it also. My patients and students have also had good results with learning self-hypnosis and using it for such suggestions to themselves at bedtime.

CONCLUSIONS

Combining hypnosis and dreamwork—especially for the majority of people who do not come by either lucid dreams or deepest trances easily— may more completely realize the interaction of primary and secondary process thought. I believe the potential therapeutic effect of this is not that primary process/"right brain," intuitive thinking is inherently wiser (although I realize there are psychology theories, especially dream theories, that do espouse exactly this idea). Rather, I believe that it is a function of how completely this mode is usually ignored, whereas logical thinking is employed ad nauseum in attempts to solve the problems of an individual's life. The primary process made need only become equally valuable in order to contribute significantly to what the rational mode has not yet achieved. And when they are working together, there is a feedback loop where the intuitive images are then evaluated by the rational process.

There may also be limited specific ways in which primary-process imagery can be uniquely beneficial by itself and for which secondary process has no equivalent: vivid emotionally connected imagery, as opposed to other forms of suggestion or ways of thinking about problems, seems to have special ability to instigate change, training waking behavior and even the body's physiological processes to follow what has just been imagined.

Hypnosis and dreams both supply this powerful rehearsal of alternative ways of being. The combination of both yields the most flexibility for directing this imagery in the direction of desired change.

REFERENCES

Albert, I., & Boone, D. (1965). Dream deprivation and facilitation with hypnosis. *Journal of Abnormal Psychology, 5,* 267–271.

Baker, E. (1983). The use of hypnotic dreaming in the treatment of the borderline patient: Some thoughts on resistance and transitional phenomena. *International Journal of Clinical and Experimental Hypnosis, 31,* 1, 19–27.

Barber, T. X. (1962). Toward a theory of hypnotic behavior: The hypnotically induced dream. *Journal of Nervous and Mental Disease, 135,* 206–221.

Barber, T. X. (1969). *Hypnosis: A scientific approach.* New York: Van Nostrand Reinhold.

Barrett, D. L. (1979a). The hypnotic dream: A content comparison to nocturnal dreams and waking fantasy. Unpublished Doctoral dissertation, University of Tennesee-Knoxville.

Barrett, D. L. (1979b). The hypnotic dream: Its content in comparison to nocturnal dreams and waking fantasy. *Journal of Abnormal Psychology, 88,* 584–591.

Barrett, D. L. (1991). Through a glass darkly: The dead appear in dreams. OMEGA: *The Journal of Death and Dying, 24,* 97–108.

Barrett, D. L. (1995). Using hypnosis to work with dreams. *Self and Society: A Journal of Humanistic Psychology, 23*(4), 25–28.

Berheim, H. (1947). *Suggestive therapeutics: A treatise on the nature and uses of hypnotism.* Translated from the French edition by C. A. Herter. New York: London Book Company.

Brady, J. P., & Rosner, B.S. (1966). Rapid eye movements in hypnotically induced dreams. *Journal of Nervous and Mental Disease, 143,* 28–35.

Brenman, M. (1949). Dreams and hypnosis. *Psychoanalytic Quarterly, 18,* 455–465.

Crasilneck, H. B., & Hall, J. A. (1975). *Clinical hypnosis: Principles and applications.* New York: Grune and Stratton, 229–230.

Dane, Joe. (1985). Comparison of waking instructions and post-hypnotic suggestions for lucid dream induction, Dissertation, Georgia State University.

Davis, L. W., & Husband, R. W. (1931). A study of hypnotic susceptibility in relation to personality traits. *Journal of Abnormal and Social Psychology, 26,* 175–182.

De Pascalis V. (1993). EEG spectral analysis during hypnotic induction, hypnotic dream and age regression. *International Journal of Psychophysiology,15*(2), 153–166.

Desoille, R. (1965). *The directed daydream.* Monograph. New York: The Psychosynthesis Research Foundation.

Domhoff, B. (1964). Night dreams and hypnotic dreams: Is there evidence that they are different? *International Journal of clinical and Experimental Hypnosis, 12,* 159–168.

Erickson, M. H. (1958). "Deep hypnosis and its induction." In L. M. LeCron (Ed.), *Experimental hypnosis.* New York: The Macmillan Company.

Fisher, C. (1953). Studies on the nature of suggestion: Part I. *Journal of the American Psychoanalytic Association, 1*, 222–255.

Fromm, Erika. (1965). Spontaneous autohypnotic age regression in a nocturnal dream. *International Journal of Clinical and Experimental Hypnosis, 13*, 119–131.

Gill, M., & Brenman, M. (1959). *Hypnosis and related states*. New York: International Universities Press.

Hall, C. S., & Van de Castle, R. L. (1966). *The content analysis of dreams*. New York: Appleton-Century-Crofts.

Hilgard, E. R. (1965). *Hypnotic susceptibility*. New York: Harcourt, Brace, & World.

Hilgard, E. R., & Nowlis, D. P. (1972). The contents of hypnotic dreams and night dreams: An exercise in methodology. In E. Fromm and R. E. Shor (Eds.), *Hypnosis: Research developments and perspectives* (pp. 85, 113). Chicago: Aldine Atherton.

Kanzer, M. (1953) The metapsychology of the hypnotic dream. *International Journal of Psychoanalysis, 34*, 228–231.

Kratochvil, S., & MacDonald, H. (1972). Sleep in hypnosis: A pilot EEG study. *American Journal of Clinical Hypnosis, 15*, 29–37.

LeCron, L. M., & Bordeaux, J. (1947). *Hypnotism today*. New York: H. Wolff, 213–214.

Mazer, M. An experimental study of the hypnotic dream. *Psychiatry, 14*, 265–277.

Mixer, B. (1961). A comparison of hypnotic and nocturnal dreams. Unpublished masters thesis, University of Missouri.

Moss, C. Scott. (1967). *The hypnotic investigation of dreams*. New York: John Wiley and Sons.

Nie, N. H. (1975). *SPSS: Statistical Package for the Social Sciences* (2nd ed.) New York: McGraw-Hill.

Sacerdote, P. (1967a). *Induced dreams*. New York: Vintage Press.

Sacerdote, P. (1967b). Therapeutic use of induced dreams. *American Journal of Clinical Hypnosis, 10*, 1–9.

Sacerdote, P. (1967b). Induced dreams: Further application. *American Journal of Clinical Hypnosis, 10*, 167–173.

Sacerdote, P. (1972). Some individualized hypnotheraputic techniques. *International Journal of Clinical and Experimental Hypnosis, 20*, 1–14.

Schiff, S., Bunney, W., & Freedman, D. (1961) A study of ocular movements in hypnotically induced dreams. *Journal of Nervous and Mental Disease, 133*, 59–67.

Schneck, J. M. (1963). Clinical and experimental aspects of hypnotic dreams. In Kline, M. V. (Ed.), *Clinical correlates of experimental hypnosis*. Springfield, IL: Thomas.

Schneck, Jerome M. (1947). The role of a dream in treatment with hypnosis. *Psychoanalytic Review, 34*, 485–491.

Schneck, J. M. (1954). Dreams in self-hypnosis. *Psychoanalytic Review, 41*, 1–8.

Schneck, J. M. (1960) Observations on the hypnotic nightmare. *American Journal of Clinical Hypnosis, 2*, 122–137.

Schneck, J. M. (1959). Self-hypnotic dreams in hypnoanalysis. *Journal of Clinical and Experimental Hypnosis, 1*, 44–53.

Schneck, J. M. (1961). The structure and function of hypnotic dreams. *Perceptual and Motor Skills, 23*, 490–497.

Schneck, J. (1974). Observations on the hypnotic nightmare. *American Journal of Clinical Hypnosis, 16*, 240–245.

Solovey, G., & Milechin, A. (1960). Hypnosis, suggestion, and oneiric activity. *American Journal of Clinical Hypnosis, 2*, 122–137.

Spanos, N. P., & Ham, M. W. (1976). Involvement in suggestion-related imaginings and the "hypnotic dream." *American Journal of Clinical Hypnosis, 18*, 43–51.

Spanos, N. P., & McPeake, J. D.(1975). Involvement in everyday imaginative activities, attitudes toward hypnosis, and hypnotic suggestibility. *Journal of Personality and Social Psychology, 31*, 594–598.

Sullivan, H. S. (1953). *The interpersonal theory of psychiatry*. New York: W. W. Norton & Company.

Sweetland, A., & Quay, H. (1952). An experimental investigation of the hypnotic dream. *Journal of Abnormal and Social Psychology, 47*, 658–682.

Tart, C. T. (1962). A comparison of suggested dreams occurring in hypnosis and sleep. *International Journal of Clinical and Experimental Hypnosis, 12*, 263–289.

Tart, C. T. (1965). The hypnotic dream: Methodological problems and a review of the literature. *Psychological Bulletin, 63*, 87–99.

Tart, C. T. (1966). Types of hypnotic dreams and their relation to hypnotic depth. *Journal of Abnormal Psychology, 71*, 377–382.

Torda, C. (1975). Dream content and anxiety and anger. *American Journal of Clinical Hypnosis, 17*, 253–259.

Walker, P. (1974). The hypnotic dream: A reconceptualization. *American Journal of Clinical Hypnosis, 16*, 246–255.

Weitzenhoffer, A. M., & Hilgard, E. R. (1962). *Stanford Hypnotic Susceptibility Scale, Form C*. Palo Alto, CA: Consulting Psychologists Press.

Zadra, A. (1996). Recurrent dreams: Their relation to life events and well-being. In D. Barrett (Ed.), *Trauma and dreams*. Boston: Harvard University Press.

Zamore, N., & Barrett, D. L. (1989) Hypnotic susceptibility and dream characteristics. *Psychiatric Journal of The University of Ottawa, 14*, 572–574.

Chapter 4

The Merits of Applying Hypnosis in the Treatment of Depression

Michael D. Yapko

OVERVIEW

Depression is a serious and already widespread problem warranting the substantial attention it receives from the mental health profession. Currently, nearly 20 million Americans are known to be suffering with the disorder, and the rate of depression in the United States is on the rise in every age group (National Institute of Mental Health, 2002). Each depressed individual directly affects many others (family, friends, co-workers), multiplying the number of people touched by depression to many tens of millions. Ultimately, we are *all* affected by depression, even if only indirectly, by having to share in the hurtful consequences of the many negative behaviors (such as drug abuse, poor parenting, and diminished productivity) that often have their origin in badly managed depression (Weissbourd, 1996).

The primary purposes of this chapter are twofold: First, to highlight some of what we already know about the nature of major depression (i.e., Major Depressive Disorder) and what seems to be effective in its treatment, and second, to draw attention to ways clinical hypnosis can further enhance aspects of the treatment process. This chapter considers the merits of hypnosis as part of a greater psychotherapy regimen for major depression only. It does not address either antidepressant medication issues or other forms of depression (such as bipolar disorder, depressed phase). When psychotherapy is clinically indicated, whether in combination with antidepressant medications or as a sole intervention, hypnosis may sensibly be employed as a means for helping facilitate the therapeutic goals. The treatment literature makes it quite clear that treatment for depression is best thought of as an active, skill-building process (Martell, Jacobson, & Addis, 2001). Hypnosis can provide a strong foundation for motivating people and empowering them with structured processes of experiential learning (Yapko, 2001, 2003, 2006). Given the reach of depression into our pockets, our personal relationships, our communities, and our very lives, addressing this complex disorder in a variety of timely and effective ways is an especially urgent challenge we as health care professionals face.

Hypnosis is not meant to be a "magical" means of suggesting that symptoms simply disappear. Rather, hypnosis is a means of absorbing people in new ways of thinking about their subjective experience, thereby potentially altering it in meaningful ways. Since the most common symptom of depression that people complain about is a sleep disturbance, after first describing general aspects of depression as a problem and hypnosis as a solution, I will focus specifically on the use of hypnosis in addressing insomnia associated with depression.

SOME OF WHAT WE KNOW ABOUT MAJOR DEPRESSION

Depression has been and continues to be heavily researched. The amount of data generated by clinicians and researchers thus far has been impressive by any standard, and has led to some firm conclusions:

- Major depression has *many* contributing factors, not a single cause. The three primary domains of the contributing factors are biological, psychological, and social. Hence, the so-called "biopsychosocial model" predominates (Cronkite & Moos, 1995; Thase & Glick, 1995).
- Depression has many underlying risk factors and a variety of comorbid conditions likely to be associated with it (Stevens, Merikangas, & Merikangas, 1995). In fact, numerous medical (e.g., cancer, heart disease) and psychological conditions (e.g., anxiety disorders, substance abuse disorders) are found to commonly coexist with depression, requiring sharp differential diagnosis and multifaceted treatment planning (American Psychiatric Association, 2000).
- Depression can be successfully managed in the majority of sufferers with medication and/or psychotherapy (Schulberg, Katon, Simon, & Rush, 1998). While no one antidepressant has definitively been shown to be superior in rates of effectiveness to another, therapeutic efficacy studies show some psychotherapies (specified later) outperform others in treating depression (Barlow, 2004).
- Medication has some treatment advantages, such as a generally faster rate of symptom remission and greater effectiveness in treating the vegetative symptoms, for example, sleep and appetite disturbances (DeBattista & Schatzberg, 1995). Medication also has some disadvantages, including uncertain dosing and effectiveness, potentially negative side effects, habituation and "poop-out" (i.e., the drug may eventually stop working), and higher initial rates of relapse (Altamura & Percudani, 1993; Dubovsky, 1997).

- Psychotherapy also has some treatment advantages and disadvantages. The therapies that enjoy the greatest empirical support are cognitive, behavioral, and interpersonal approaches (Depression Guideline Panel, 1993). The advantages include therapy's focus on skill building and the associated reduced relapse rate, the value of the therapeutic relationship, the greater degree of personal empowerment, and the potential to not just perform a "mop up" of preexisting problems but to instead teach the skills of *prevention* (Seligman, 1990; Yapko, 1999). The disadvantages of psychotherapy include the greater reliance on the level of clinician competence (i.e., experience and judgment), the greater time lag between the initiation of treatment and the remission of symptoms compared to medications, the lesser effect in reducing vegetative symptoms, and the potential detrimental side effects of client exposure to a clinician's particular theoretical or philosophical stance (Mondimore,1993; Thase & Howland, 1995).
- The extraordinary ongoing success of the Human Genome Project has highlighted the complex relationship between genetics, environment, and specific disorders. Genetic vulnerabilities or predispositions exist, but they operate in association with environmental variables that may increase or decrease their likelihood of expression (Siever, 1997). In the specific case of (unipolar) major depression, the genetic contribution has been shown to be significant, with environmental factors (both social and psychological) appearing to also have significant influence in its onset (Kaelber, Moul, & Farmer, 1995). (In contrast, the genetic component of bipolar disorder has been shown to be a strong one; Dubovsky, 1997.) The relationship between neurochemicals and experience is bidirectional, meaning environmental triggers influence neurochemistry *at least* as much as neurochemistry influences experience (Azar, 1997; Dubovsky, 1997; Siever, 1997). There is evidence to suggest that psychotherapy may be a means for directly and/or indirectly affecting neurotransmitter levels in the brain, perhaps in some a parallel to the effects of medication (Schwartz & Begley, 2002).

Research has yielded many other insights about depression, of course, but the previous statements reflect a high level of general consensus among depression experts.

Some of What We Know about Treating Depression with Psychotherapy

Depression isn't just "suggested away" with hypnotic suggestions. Hypnosis has to be employed realistically by aiming at and modifying appropriate targets in treatment. Thus, this section will discuss some of what seems to matter most in clinical intervention.

A number of important insights about major depression and suggestions for its treatment were articulated in the depression treatment guidelines developed by the United States Agency for Health Care Policy and Research (AHCPR), now the Agency for Healthcare Quality and Research (AHQR; Depression Guideline Panel, 1993): (1) Three psychotherapies were shown to have the greatest amount of empirical support—cognitive, behavioral, and interpersonal psychotherapies. These are identified as the psychotherapies of choice, and any or all can be applied *according to the client's symptom profile* (*not* the clinician's preferred orientation); (2) Psychotherapy should be an *active* process in the way it is conducted, involving active exchanges between clinician and client that would typically involve providing psychoeducation, the development of skill-building strategies, the use of homework assignments, and the use of the therapy relationship as both a foundation and a vehicle for exploring relevant ideas and perspectives; (3) Therapy should not only focus on problem solving, but the teaching of problem-solving skills, especially as they relate to symptom resolution, the guidelines' suggested focus of treatment; (4) Effective therapy need not have an historical focus. According to the treatment guidelines, the most effective therapies are goal-oriented, skill-building approaches. *None* of them focus on attaining extensive historical data to explain the origins of depression. Rather, they focus on developing solutions to problems and coping skills for managing symptoms. Hypnosis is especially amenable to each of these psychotherapeutic applications, since it, too, is an active and directive means of intervention. The same indications and contraindications as articulated in the treatment guidelines (Depression Guideline Panel, 1993) prevail when applying hypnosis, particularly the recommendation that clinicians adapt their approach according to the patient's symptom profile rather than a specific theoretical allegiance.

In performing an extensive review of clinical and research literature in order to prepare the depression treatment guidelines, the panel formed the conclusion that trying to find a specific origin for an individual's depression was unnecessary in promoting recovery. This sharply distinguishes what might be termed an *event-driven* perspective (the view that depression has its origin in specific historical events that must be identified and "worked through") from what could be called a *process-driven* perspective (the view that depression has its roots in ongoing ways of erroneously or negatively interpreting or managing various life experiences). Recognizing that depression arises for *many* reasons of a process-driven nature accentuates the realization that *by the time depression strikes most individuals, one or more risk factors* (such as perceptual style, cognitive style, and level of social and problem-solving skills) *had already been well in place* (Seligman, 1989).

The research makes it abundantly clear that depression is much more than a biologically based problem (Joiner, Coyne, & Blalock, 1999; Yapko, 2006). Thus, helping people recognize that depression arises, in part, because of social and psychological factors can help them to avail themselves of the benefits psychotherapy can provide. After all, no amount of medication (or brain stimulation or brainwave reeducation) can provide people with better problem-solving skills, coping skills, cognitive skills, relationship skills, or a supportive network of friends. Of the various approaches to treating depression that have been evaluated scientifically, there is unequivocal evidence that the therapies that actively encourage people to develop specific life-enhancing skills perform better than other therapies that do not (Martell et al., 2001).

As our understandings of both hypnosis and depression have deepened in recent years, the antiquated concerns that hypnosis would hurt rather than help the depressed client have markedly diminished. We have learned, for example, that suicidality isn't about "inadequate ego defenses," and that depression isn't really about "anger turned inward." Instead, we have learned that there are specific risk factors evident in one's thinking, behaving, relating, and perceiving that can, under certain stressful conditions, give rise to depressive episodes. As a result, there are many more immediate and well-defined targets for hypnotic intervention than previously realized. It has been amply demonstrated that psychotherapy can succeed, and succeed well, when people who suffer depression are taught key life skills that empower them to live more personally satisfying lives.

One can describe the term *depression* as a global shorthand, a convenient label for a wide range of symptoms and patterns of experience. Effective treatment must first involve identifying the salient patterns that regulate the experience of depression in a given individual. We also know that therapy, *any* therapy, will necessarily have to interrupt ongoing patterns of experience in some way and generate some new patterns of experience that prove beneficial to the client's mood, outlook, and behavior. The task for the clinician is to *absorb* the client in new patterns, whether patterns of thought as in cognitive therapy, patterns of physiology as in somatic-based interventions, or whatever patterns are addressed in a specific style of intervention. Hypnosis is multidimensional in its ability to focus anywhere and catalyze the merits of the intervention, whatever form it might take.

As stated earlier, depression is the product of many contributing variables. Can hypnosis be used in ways that address risk factors and the process underlying the formation of some forms of depression? This chapter offers both evidence and clinical experience in using hypnosis in just such a manner.

THE EMPIRICAL BASIS FOR EMPLOYING HYPNOSIS IN THE TREATMENT OF DEPRESSION

The body of literature describing the relationship between the quality of one's beliefs and one's mood is substantial. It is well established that the positive, optimistic person is less likely to suffer depression. Likewise, such a person will also benefit: (1) *physically* by likely suffering less serious illness and higher rates of recovery; (2) in terms of *productivity*, having higher levels of focus, persistence, and frustration tolerance; and, (3) in terms of greater *sociability* and likeability, enjoying the many health and mood benefits associated with having more close and positive relationships (Peterson, 2000; Seligman, 1989, 1990, 2000; Yapko, 1997, 1999, 2001).

The overlap between depression as a problem and hypnosis as a means for addressing it centers on the "believed-in imaginations" of the depressed client. Believing "life is unfair," or "I'm no good," or "I'll never be able to do that" are just a very few of the many self-limiting and even self-injurious beliefs that depressed individuals may form and come to hold as true. Thus, it is no coincidence that cognitive-behavioral therapies, which challenge depressed individuals to learn how to identify and self-correct their cognitive distortions and behave more effectively, have been shown to be highly effective approaches (Clarkin, Pilkonis, & Magrude,1996; Greenberger & Padesky, 1995).

It is terribly unfortunate that the scientific literature about the use of hypnosis specifically with depressed populations is sparse because of how long hypnosis was discouraged as a treatment tool based on misinformation discussed earlier. However, that is beginning to change; in a recent book edited by the author of this chapter (Yapko, 2006), many well-known clinicians and hypnosis experts described their applications of hypnosis in a variety of clinical populations all sharing an underlying depression.

A variety of therapeutic efficacy studies have been published attesting to the added value of hypnosis to established treatments, especially cognitive-behavioral approaches (Lynn, Kirsch, Barabasz, Cardena, & Patterson, 2000; Kirsch, Montgomery, & Sapirstein, 1995; Schoenberger, 2000.) In one recent study of hypnosis applied specifically to a depressed population (Alladin & Alibhai, 2007), the group receiving hypnosis treatments in combination with cognitive behavioral therapy (CBT) showed greater reduction in depression, anxiety, and hopelessness than the group receiving CBT alone. Depression is a global term, however. In fact, depression is comprised of many different components, including cognitive patterns (such as attributional style), behavioral patterns (such as avoidant coping styles), and relational patterns (such as hypercriticalness). Many of these components have been addressed successfully with hypnosis (Kirsch, 1996; Schoenberger, 2000; Schoenberger, Kirsch, Gearan, Montgomery, & Pastyrnak, 1997). Employing these treatments with depressed populations for whom these cognitive and behavioral issues would be relevant would undoubtedly improve their condition. In fact, much of what is presented in this chapter could be characterized as cognitive-behavioral therapy performed within a hypnotic and strategic framework (Yapko, 1988, 1992, 1993, 2006).

WHAT IS POSSIBLE IN HYPNOSIS?

The fact that people can manifest a variety of normally "hidden" capacities in hypnosis is the reason why hypnosis offers so much as a treatment tool. If one were to do even a cursory review of the scientific literature attesting to the value of hypnosis in a variety of medical, dental, psychotherapeutic, and educational settings, one would find an enormous array of high-quality research that supports its use. More recently, newer technologies for conducting brain scans (i.e., fMRI, CAT, PET, and SPECT) have spawned new insights into the working relationship between the mind and brain. Similarly, using advanced diagnostic tools to affirm measurable changes in physiology in response to "mere" suggestions (such as influencing blood flow, muscular tension, immunological responses, and perceptions of pain) has led to a virtual explosion of applications of hypnosis in behavioral medicine.

In hypnosis, people are able to manifest a variety of talents that are collectively termed "hypnotic phenomena." These include: (1) *age regression* (defined as the intense and experiential absorption in memory such that memories can be recalled in vivid detail and perhaps even relived as if occurring in the now, allowing for the reframing of memories, for example); (2) *age progression* (defined as the intense and experiential absorption in expectations, a vehicle for establishing positive self-fulfilling prophecies, for example); (3) *analgesia and anesthesia* (the ability to reduce or even eliminate sensation, exceptionally valuable in the treatment of all kinds of pain); and (4) *dissociation* (the ability to break global experiences into component parts and selectively amplify or de-amplify a part depending on therapeutic objective, such as encouraging a controlled detachment from overwhelming emotions). There are many other hypnotic phenomena that become accessible in hypnosis that are also beneficial to employ in the course of psychotherapy, and the interested reader may choose to learn more than this brief chapter can address. Suffice it to say that as one considers what is possible in hypnosis, *wherever one can influence mental or physical processes* it quickly becomes apparent that, the limits of which have not been anywhere even close to defined yet, *hypnosis will be valuable.*

WAYS TO USE HYPNOSIS IN PSYCHOTHERAPY

A clinician has to be deliberate about choosing focal points for his or her interventions. Focusing on someone's cognitions, for example, shouldn't be a standard procedure as a self-identified cognitive therapist. Rather, it should be a choice one makes to focus on the client's thoughts because there is a powerful depressogenic pattern operating on that dimension. But, for someone else, the focus will need to be on his or her relationships, and for someone else on his or her sleep difficulties. What a clinician will focus on and amplify with hypnosis will, hopefully, differ according to the unique profile of each individual client. This is one of the great strengths of being knowledgeable about hypnosis: *the ability to make good therapeutic choices based on client need outweighs loyalty to a particular theory of intervention.*

There are many different ways to apply hypnosis in psychotherapy. Since hypnosis is not generally considered a therapy in its own right, hypnosis is typically integrated with other psychotherapeutic treatments, such as cognitive-behavioral therapy (CBT) or interpersonal therapy (IPT). Thus, how one applies hypnosis will be entirely consistent with however one thinks about the nature of peoples' symptoms and the nature of therapeutic intervention.

Hypnosis essentially amplifies experience. So, if one wants to focus the client on his or her cognitive dimension of experience, perhaps to teach a client to recognize and correct so-called cognitive distortions, one might use hypnosis to help make such identification and correction a more natural and even more automatic process. (Aaron Beck, a founding father of modern cognitive therapy, may not talk about "the unconscious" the way a hypnosis practitioner might, but he speaks readily of "automatic thoughts." What about hypnosis to instill *positive* automatic thoughts?)

Hypnosis can be used to help *manage symptoms*. This is a more superficial, yet meaningful, application of hypnosis. Using hypnosis to reduce anxiety or rumination so an anxious or depressed client can enhance his or her sleep, for example, is not a "deep" intervention, yet clinically it is an enormously valuable one (Yapko, 2006). Teaching someone to manage pain is not psychologically "deep," but can literally save peoples' lives (Phillips, 2006).

Hypnosis can be used to *foster skill acquisition*. As alluded to before, teaching clients specific skills (e.g., social skills or problem-solving skills) is a standard part of almost any therapy. It is well established that experiential learning is the most powerful form of learning. Hypnosis is a vehicle of experiential learning. It's not just something to consider or distantly imagine. It's something to be absorbed on many different levels. There is plenty of evidence that hypnosis generally enhances psychotherapy for this very reason. Thus, when comparing CBT without hypnosis versus CBT with hypnosis, the addition of the hypnosis enhances therapeutic efficacy. (Note that the salient research question is not how hypnosis compares to CBT, but how CBT *without* compares to CBT *with* hypnosis.)

Hypnosis can be used to *establish associations and dissociations*. What aspect(s) of experience do we want the client more connected or associated to? What aspect(s) of experience do we want the client disconnected or dissociated from? Someone who is lacking emotional awareness (what might be termed "affective dissociation" in hypnotic terms) can benefit from an emotionally focused (associative) intervention, while someone who is hyperemotional (emotionally associative) might benefit from a more cognitively based (emotionally dissociative) intervention. Hypnosis allows one to structure interventions according to whatever aspects of experience might best serve the client to associate to or dissociate from (or to amplify or de-amplify). And, if one thinks in these terms, it is easy to see how *any* therapy similarly focuses on or away from specific dimensions of experience, though predictably less effectively by not using the amplified experience of the hypnotic condition.

Hypnosis is regarded as a tool, a vehicle for dispensing information, building perspective, enhancing skill acquisition, and creating a context for therapeutic change to take place. Thus, one can use hypnosis to highlight to a patient his or her cognitive distortions, offering suggestions for more automatically recognizing and refuting them. Thus, if one wishes to make use of cognitive therapy techniques, hypnosis can be used to help establish therapeutic associations in the patient for more readily identifying and clarifying his or her distorted thoughts and attributions (Yapko, 1992, 2003).

Similarly, if one chooses to focus on the relational dimension, using an interpersonal model as a conceptual and practical framework, hypnosis is also applicable. Identifying and relating skillfully to other peoples' needs and values, establishing and consistently enforcing one's limits in one's dealings with others, and developing greater awareness of one's own needs and how they might best be met are all examples of skills one might wish to help the patient build using hypnotic suggestions.

In short, the ability of hypnosis, applied either formally or informally, to build a strong link between the troublesome context and the skilled response desired in that context is the primary reason why hypnosis can be so easily integrated into virtually any model of treatment.

There are many other ways to use hypnosis—to build positive expectations, to amplify and work with emotion-laden memories, to enhance cognitive flexibility, to instill better coping skills, and to increase self-efficacy are just a few applications immediately relevant to a sophisticated therapy practice, regardless of one's preferred theoretical orientation.

WHAT MAKES HYPNOSIS VALUABLE IN THE TREATMENT OF DEPRESSION?

Hypnosis may be valuable in treatment because of its relationship to subjective states like depression. Upon deeper reflection, the overlaps between the separate yet related domains of hypnosis and depression become more evident. I'll describe just a few of these: (1) Both come about and increase in intensity the more narrow your focus; (2) Both are ultimately social processes, greatly influenced by your relationships with others, whether the other is a clinical authority describing the therapeutic merits of exposing you to an induction procedure, or the other is a parent or spouse describing the flaws in your character; (3) Both are a product of expectancy, whether the expectation is one of getting the benevolent corrective message "into your unconscious" through suggestions received in a dissociated state, or whether the expectation is that no amount of your effort will result in a success, thereby giving rise to the apathy so typical of depression; and (4) Both involve what hypnosis pioneers Theodore Sarbin and, later, Ernest Hilgard, described when they suggested hypnosis is, in part, a "believed-in imagination," an experience based on the recognition that people can and do get deeply absorbed in

highly subjective beliefs and perceptions that quite literally regulate the quality of their lives (Sarbin, 1997; Hilgard, personal communication, 1988).
These beliefs and perceptions can be altered and amplified during the experience of hypnosis, well illustrating the point how idiosyncratic each person's
sense of reality really is, especially in response to "mere" suggestions.

The notion of an individual's personal reality essentially being a "believed-
in imagination" preceded the origin and development of cognitive therapy by
decades, even centuries, and firmly established the relevance of hypnosis in
treatment. Cognitive-behavioral therapy is, at this time, probably the most
well-researched method of therapeutic intervention. It is founded on the premise that people in general, and depressed people in particular, regularly
make identifiable errors in information processing, thinking and genuinely
believing in their mistaken notions of what truly—and depressingly—seems
like reality to them (Beck, 1997; Beck, Rush, Shaw, & Emery, 1979). This
process of becoming absorbed in one's (depressing) imaginings is, indeed, an
instructive parallel to what occurs in hypnosis, where a clinician performs an
induction and attempts to absorb the individual in alternative ways of experiencing him or herself.

Through procedures employing hypnosis, the clinician creates a context
where the individual can change the direction and quality of his or her focus.
Perhaps the suggested focus is on engaging in some new life-enhancing
behavior, or perhaps on exciting and motivating glimpses of future possibilities, or possibly on rewriting some of the negative internal dialogue, or some-
how altering for the better any of literally scores of depressing focal points
(e.g., cognitive styles, coping styles, relational styles). What the clinician suggests during hypnosis may not be any more true in an objective sense than
what the person previously believed—it may just feel much better and serve
the person better. Hypnosis as a means of teaching people, a vehicle for getting new possibilities for thinking, feeling, behaving, and relating integrated
more quickly and deeply is precisely why knowledgeable clinicians do hypnosis in the first place.

HYPNOSIS AND POSITIVE PSYCHOLOGY

With an increasing emphasis within the psychotherapy profession to pay
more attention to what's *right* with people rather than what's wrong with
them (Seligman, 2000), the very first lesson one learns when studying hypnosis takes on a new significance: What you focus on you amplify. Do we as
mental health professionals want to focus on pathology or wellness? Is the
goal of treatment to decrease pathology or weakness, or to expand strength?
These are not merely semantic issues. On the contrary, how one responds to
a client's distress and organizes therapeutic intervention is broadly based on
whether one strives to identify and address client weaknesses or strengths.

In this sense, hypnosis can be thought of as the original positive psychology. Indeed, well before the term *positive psychology* was coined in just the last decade, pioneering psychiatrist Milton H. Erickson, MD, as early as the 1940s, was writing about the need to pay more attention to and thereby amplify peoples' strengths. Erickson is often described as the most creative and influential clinician (as opposed to theorist) of the twentieth century, and it is hardly a coincidence that so many of his innovative contributions directly involved insightful applications of clinical hypnosis (Haley, 1973; Zeig, 1980).

Anyone who practices clinical hypnosis does so with the firmly entrenched and therapeutically invaluable belief that people have many more abilities than they consciously realize. Hypnosis engenders an entirely optimistic appraisal of people such that therapy gets organized around the belief that people can discover and develop the very resources within themselves they need to improve. Hypnosis creates an amplified, energized, high-powered context for people to explore, discover, and use more of their innate abilities. *Hypnosis isn't the therapy, and hypnosis itself cures nothing.* Rather, hypnosis is the vehicle for empowering people with the abilities and realizations that ultimately serve to help them. It isn't the experience of hypnosis itself that's therapeutic, it's what happens *during* hypnosis in terms of developing new and helpful associations. The study of hypnosis, then, involves a process of discovering what latent capacities are accessible in the experience of hypnosis, and how to bring them forth at the times and places they will best serve the client. It truly is a positive psychology in practice.

HYPNOSIS AND BUILDING REALISTIC EXPECTANCY

One of the strongest factors contributing to the viability of hypnosis as an intervention tool is termed "expectancy" (Coe, 1993; Kirsch, 2000). Expectancy refers to that quality of the client's belief system that leads him or her to believe that the procedure implemented by the clinician will produce a therapeutic result. Positive expectancy for treatment involves multiple perceptions: The clinician is seen as credible and benevolent, the procedure seems to have a plausible perhaps even compelling rationale, and the therapy context itself seems to support its application. Thus, by the client being instructed in the value and the methods of hypnosis, whether directly or indirectly, an expectation is established that the associated procedures will have some potentially therapeutic benefit, increasing the likelihood of them actually doing so (Barber, 1991; Zeig, 1980).

Expectancy is an especially critical issue in the treatment of major depression. Cognitive theory in particular has viewed depression as existing on a three-point foundation of negative expectations, negative interpretation of events, and negative self-evaluation (Beck, Rush, Shaw, & Emery, 1979). An individual's negative expectancy for life experience is a cognitive pattern and risk factor that has been associated with difficulties not only in the realm of mood, but also in poorer physical health, poorer social adjustment, and diminished productivity. Furthermore, negative expectancy has been associated to lowered treatment success rates (Seligman, 1989, 1990). At the extreme, negative expectancy in the form of a pervasive sense of hopelessness can be associated with suicidality (Beck, Brown, Berchick, Stewart, & Steer, 1990). Establishing positive expectancy in a variety of specific contexts may be a necessary ingredient in effective treatment (Yapko, 1988, 1992, 1993, 2001). Age progression in hypnosis as a vehicle for concretely establishing a positive and motivating view of the future may be helpful in this regard (Torem, 1987, 1992, 2006; Yapko, 1988, 1992, 2001, 2003, 2006).

Important as it may be, however, a focus on expectancy to the exclusion of other factors of potential therapeutic effectiveness can also be limiting. Someone can have positive expectations yet generate no meaningful therapeutic results for a variety of reasons. For every client who began therapy with high hopes that went unfulfilled, the point is clear that positive expectations are not enough. They must be realistic and they must occur within a larger therapeutic framework that is able to convert the promise of expectancy into the reality of a goal accomplished. Expectancy matters, but even positive, well-defined expectations can become a source of problems rather than a source of solutions if they are unrealistic. Thus, a clinician must be able to educate the client in the process of distinguishing realistic from unrealistic expectations, whether positive *or* negative. Hypnosis can help in this therapeutic endeavor.

TARGETING THE MOST COMMON SYMPTOM OF DEPRESSION: HYPNOSIS AND PSYCHOTHERAPY FOR INSOMNIA

The time hypnosis may be of greatest benefit in psychotherapy is when it is used as a means of teaching skills that can empower the therapy client (Yapko, 2001, 2003). Regarding insomnia in particular, the most common symptom of depression, there are a number of specific skills that someone suffering insomnia can learn that will make a positive difference, such as relaxation and good sleep hygiene. However, there is another specific skill that is an amenable target for a well-crafted hypnotic intervention. That target is called "rumination."

Rumination is the cognitive process of spinning around the same thoughts over and over again. It is considered an enduring style of coping with ongoing problems and stressors, a coping style that can both lead to and exacerbate depression. One's coping style is a significant factor in one's overall mental health and is an especially important factor in depression. Although coping responses may be classified in many ways, most approaches distinguish between strategies oriented toward confronting the problem and strategies oriented toward reducing tension by avoiding dealing with the problem directly (Holahan, Moos, & Bonin, 1999). Rumination can be thought of as a pattern of avoidance that actually increases anxiety and agitation. Ruminative responses include repeatedly expressing to others how badly one feels, pondering to excess why one feels bad, and catastrophizing the negative effects of feeling bad (Nolen-Hoeksema, 1991.) By ruminating, the person avoids having to take decisive and timely action, further compounding a personal sense of inadequacy. Rumination leads to more negative interpretations of life events, greater recall of negative autobiographical memories and events, impaired problem solving, and a reduced willingness to participate in pleasant activities (Spasojević & Alloy, 2001). As Just & Alloy (1997) stated, correlational, field, longitudinal, and experimental studies all provide evidence that ruminative behavior is not only highly associated with depression, but serves to increase both the severity and duration of episodes of depression. The common term *analysis paralysis* describes the hazard of ruminating at the expense of taking effective action.

It is especially significant that rumination not only features in the quality of one's depression, but it actually *predicts* depression. Susan Nolen-Hoeksema of Yale University published enormously valuable research that establishes the link clearly: A ruminative coping style that precedes depressive symptoms predicts higher levels of depressive symptoms over time (after accounting for baseline levels), onset of new depressive disorders, greater chronicity of depressive disorders, and higher levels of anxiety symptoms (Nolen-Hoeksema, 2000, 2003).

Thus, rumination is an especially high-priority target at which to aim one's interventions, hypnotic or otherwise. Rumination generates both somatic and cognitive arousal, both of which can exacerbate insomnia, but the evidence suggests cognitive arousal is the greater problem. As Harvey (2000) reported in her research on the relationship between cognitive arousal and insomnia, insomniacs were *ten* times more likely to cite cognitive arousal as central to their sleep difficulties, compared with somatic arousal. Harvey went on to say that the need to aim for minimal cognitive processing and effort toward sleep are key treatment goals.

HYPNOSIS, TARGETING RUMINATION AND ENHANCING SLEEP

Having asked literally hundreds of individuals who declare themselves "good sleepers" what they tend to think about when they go to sleep, their common and consistent answer is some variation of the reply, "nothing." That doesn't mean literally that they think of nothing and have an "empty mind." Rather, it means that the content of what they think about is so simple and nonthreatening that it generates no significant somatic or cognitive arousal to interfere with sleep. Conversely, when I ask people who say they sleep poorly what they think about when going to sleep, they typically say some variation of, "everything." They think of worrisome problems, unresolved situations needing to be addressed, obligations to be met, tasks still needing to be done, and on and on. The levels of cognitive and somatic arousal are raised to the point of interfering with sleep.

The use of hypnosis to teach the ability to direct one's own thoughts rather than merely react to them is a well-established dynamic and a principal reason for employing hypnosis in any context (Lynn & Kirsch, 2006; Yapko, 2003). Reducing the stressful wanderings of an agitated mind and also relaxing the body while simultaneously helping people create and follow a line of pleasant thoughts and images that can soothe and calm the person are valuable goals in the service of enhancing sleep.

In order to achieve these aims, there are a number of important components to include in one's treatment plan. These include: (1) Teaching the client how to efficiently distinguish between useful analysis and useless ruminations. The distinction features variations in factors such as the amount of research, if any, to be done and the timing of a decision to act (i.e., how much information to gather and how long to contemplate what to do), but the single most important distinguishing characteristic is the conversion from analysis to action; (2) Enhancing skills in compartmentalization in order to better separate bedtime from problem-solving time with the well-defined goal in place of keeping them separate; (3) Establishing better coping skills that involve more direct and effective problem-solving strategies. For the client that avoids making decisions and implementing them out of the fear of making the wrong one, such as perfectionist individuals, who are also at higher risk for depression as a result of their perfectionism (Basco, 1999), he or she will need additional help learning to make sensible and effective, albeit sometimes imperfect, problem-solving decisions; (4) Helping the client develop effective strategies for choosing among a range of alternatives. There is evidence that having more options, an oft-stated goal for clinicians, actually increases the anxiety and depression of those who don't have a good strategy for choosing among many alternatives (Schwartz, 2004); (5) addressing issues of sleep hygiene and attitudes toward sleep in order to make sure the person's behavior and attitudes are consistent with good sleep; and (6) Teaching "mind-clearing" or "mind-focusing" strategies, especially self-hypnosis strategies of one type or another that help the person direct their thinking in utterly benign directions.

Each of the first five components listed here support the potential value of the sixth, the actual hypnosis strategy one employs to help calm the person to sleep.

HYPNOTIC APPROACHES

Hypnosis can be used as a vehicle for teaching the client effective ways to make distinctions between useful analysis and useless ruminations, compartmentalize various aspects of experience, develop better coping skills, develop more effective decision-making strategies, and develop good behavioral and thought habits regarding sleep. Such hypnosis sessions are quite different in their structure than is a session designed specifically for the purpose of enhancing the ability to fall and stay asleep.

The primary difference between a sleep session and a regular therapy session employing hypnosis is that hypnosis for sleep enhancement is designed to actually lead the client to fall asleep. In standard therapy sessions involving hypnosis, the opposite is true—the clinician takes active steps to prevent the client from falling asleep during the session. It has been well established that hypnosis isn't a sleep state, and that sleep learning is a myth. Thus, clinicians employing hypnosis encourage the client to become focused, relaxed, yet maintain a sufficient degree of alertness to be capable of participating in the session by listening and actively adapting the clinician's suggestions to his or her particular needs.

Another key difference between a hypnosis session for enhancing sleep and a standard therapy session is the role of the client during the process. In therapy, the client is defined as an active participant—actively involved in the search for relevance for the clinician's suggestions, actively involved in absorbing and integrating the suggestions, and actively finding ways to apply them in the service of self-help. Relaxation may or may not be a part of the process. In fact, some suggestions a clinician offers during hypnosis might even be anxiety provoking or challenging to the client's sense of comfort. After all, personal growth often means stepping outside one's "comfort zone." In the sleep session, however, cognitive and somatic arousal are to be minimized, and so challenges to the client's beliefs (or expectations, role definition, or any other aspect a clinician might appropriately challenge) are precluded.

The content of the strategy (e.g., progressive relaxation, imagery from a favorite place, recollection of a happy memory, creation of fantasy stories, counting sheep, etc.) is a secondary consideration. Thus, what specific hypnotic approach one uses is relatively unimportant. The primary consideration is that whatever the person focuses on, it needs to be something that reduces both somatic and cognitive arousal.

Approaches can be direct or indirect according to what the client finds easiest to respond to. Likewise, they can be content or process oriented, again depending on what the client finds easiest to relate to. Since sleep isn't something that can be commanded, an authoritarian style is generally counterproductive. A permissive style is both gentler and more consistent with an attitude of allowing sleep to occur instead of trying to force it to occur.

The use of recorded hypnotic approaches (i.e., tape recordings or compact disc recordings) can be a useful means of helping the client to develop the skills in focusing on calming suggestions. Generally, these should be considered a temporary help in the process so that the person is eventually able to fall and stay asleep independently using self-hypnosis. However, recordings pose no major or even minor hazards that warrant concern they will be abused in some way, so there seems to be no good reason to push clients to stop using the recordings for as long as they find them helpful.

Helping people learn to "slow down," curtail their ruminations, establish stronger boundaries between their work and personal lives, and better separate problem-solving time from sleep time are all worthwhile goals to address in treatment. These are life skills that may be learned with clinicians serving as teachers or guides. Hypnosis can be an effective vehicle for teaching such skills, even if just teaching basic relaxation skills, perhaps even outperforming sleep medications. As one prominent sleep and depression researcher wrote, "using deep muscle relaxation and other forms of progressive relaxation strategies may help individuals to fall asleep more quickly . . . controlled studies suggest effects as strong as, and with greater durability than, those observed with sedative hypnotics" (Thase, 2000, pp. 49–50). The quality of the symptoms a client presents can point the clinician in the direction he or she might go if the client is to be sufficiently empowered to get some control back and reduce or eliminate symptoms. *For as long as a client feels victimized by his or her symptoms, recovery from depression is extremely unlikely* (Cohen, 1994).

The goals of therapy include not only reducing or eliminating symptoms, but also reducing or eliminating associated risk factors for further episodes. Depression is often described in the literature as a "recurrent disease," and relapse statistics confirm an ever-higher probability of later episodes the more episodes one has (Glass, 1999). Using the previous example of insomnia as a target, insomnia is the symptom. But, unless the individual's ruminative coping style is altered, and unless the person's global cognitive style is addressed by teaching better compartmentalization (boundary) skills (e.g., to separate problem-solving time from sleep time), the mere teaching of relaxation skills is unlikely to be of enough help to the person to overcome depression.

A SAMPLE TRANSCRIPT OF HYPNOTIC SUGGESTIONS TO ENHANCE SLEEP

The following abbreviated hypnosis transcript can illustrate what kinds of suggestions might be given to someone who tends to ruminate at bedtime. The goal is to provide a comfortable, relaxed experience in which the person discovers he or she can clear his or her mind of the "clutter" that interferes with sleep.

I'd like to invite you to arrange yourself in a position that is comfortable. I'd encourage you to listen to the recording of this session while you are lying in bed so you can drift off to sleep and then sleep comfortably through the night. Unlike other kinds of sessions we've done involving hypnosis or relaxation processes, with this particular hypnosis session it *is* appropriate for you to listen to it while you're in bed as you're going to sleep. After all, the purpose of this particular session is to make your sleep easier, more satisfying, and more restful.

So, with that in mind, I'd like you to let your eyes close . . . and notice the differences instantly as soon as you let your eyes close . . . It means you are no longer focusing on things around you. . it means that you have closed your eyes to the outside world . . . for now . . . And in a way . . . you might think of that . . . simple action of closing your eyes . . . as starting to close out . . . the world out there . . . Now, certainly you'll hear . . . the sounds . . . the routine sounds . . . of your environment . . . and because they are so routine . . . whether it is a dog barking or crickets chirping . . . or traffic . . . it doesn't matter what it is . . . it's routine . . . And that frees your mind . . . to be very present in this moment which precedes your sleep . . . you get to let your mind . . . grow ever quieter . . . ever more comfortable . . . and notice how good that feels . . . It's really quite soothing to now recognize that you can . . . slowly turn down . . . the rate and volume of your thoughts . . . until you find yourself . . . thinking in a slow, quiet whisper . . . that is barely audible . . . and what matters is that you have the ability . . . to focus your thoughts on whatever soothes you . . . and relaxes you . . . and makes you feel good . . . there's so much freedom in just relaxing and not having to think . . . you can feel the freedom . . . of being able to . . . drift off . . . to sleep . . . slowly . . . deliberately . . . And, little by little . . . you may become aware . . . that you really aren't thinking about anything in particular . . . and how your attention stays ever more focused on . . . the wonderfully . . . comfortable . . . immediacy . . . of the safety and warmth . . . the deeply comfortable warmth . . . of your bed . . . And then you can notice the subtle sensations . . . associated with falling asleep . . . Which parts of your body . . . seem to drift off . . . first? . . . Which parts are heaviest . . . as if it would take just massive effort to move them? . . . And which parts are lightest . . . and free . . . And with your breathing slowing . . . and your mind . . . growing ever quieter . . . it can feel wonderful . . . to be drifting off . . . so easily . . . and effortlessly . . . and there's no need to drift off to sleep just yet . . . unless you really want to . . . but you can allow yourself . . . the luxury . . . of being in this . . . state of mind . . . and body . . . for a long restful time . . . And when you wake up after this deep, restful sleep . . . many hours from now . . . you'll naturally feel rested . . . and energized . . . it's a powerful experience . . . of rediscovering . . . quite

naturally . . . that you can sleep . . . you can sleep . . . deeply . . . And
so you can . . . just enjoy . . . the comfort . . . the sense of peacefulness
. . . that you can carry with you into your dreams . . . and sleep . . . sleep
. . . So now . . . you can drift off . . . drift off . . . and sleep well . . . Good
night.

CONCLUSION

It is no coincidence that of the therapies with the greatest level of empirical support for their effectiveness in treating depression (cognitive-
behavioral and interpersonal), *none of them* focus on the past and *all of them*
focus on helping depression sufferers build the skills that can empower them.
In this chapter, I have emphasized the merits of hypnosis as a vehicle for
teaching new skills, encouraging active experimentation with them in everyday contexts, and using the feedback from life experience to continually
adapt oneself to changing demands. Such teachings directly counter the
popular psychologies that emphasize non-discriminately "trusting your guts"
or "living in the present" or thinking "you can have it all" and countless
other such global phrases that set people up to get hurt when they discover
the hard way these principles don't apply in all (or perhaps even most) life
situations.

Hypnosis can reasonably be considered the original "positive psychology."
Anyone who applies hypnosis does so with the firm belief that people have
more resources than they consciously realize, and that hypnosis can help
bring these resources to the fore. Empowering people in this way is a natural
component of an effective treatment for depression, for no one can overcome depression while feeling or behaving in a disempowered manner.
Hopefully, as we continue to learn more about the many pathways into
depression, we will learn more about the many pathways out as well, including those involving skillful applications of hypnosis.

REFERENCES

Alladin, A., & Alibhai, A. (2007). Cognitive hypnotherapy for depression: An em-
      pirical investigation. *International Journal of Clinical and Experimental Hypnosis*,
      55(2), 147–166.
Altamura, A., & Percudani, M. (1993). The use of antidepressants for long-term
      treatment of recurrent depression: Rationale, current methodologies, and
      future directions. *Journal of Clinical Psychiatry*, 54 (8, supplement), 1–23.
American Psychiatric Association. (2000). *Diagnostic and statistical manual (4th edition,
      revised)*. Washington, D.C.: American Psychiatric Association.
Azar, B. (April, 1997). Environment is key to serotonin levels. *APA Monitor, 28*,
      4, 26–29.

Barber, J. (1991). The locksmith model: Accessing hypnotic responsiveness. In S. Lynn & J. Rhue (Eds.), *Theories of hypnosis: Current models and perspectives* (pp. 241–274). New York: Guilford.

Barlow, D. (2004). Psychological treatments. *American Psychologist, 59*(9), 869–878.

Basco, M. (1999). *Never good enough: Freeing yourself from the chains of perfectionism.* New York: Simon & Schuster.

Beck, A. (1997). Cognitive therapy: Reflections. In J. Zeig (Ed.), *The evolution of psychotherapy: The third conference* (pp. 55–64). New York: Brunner/Mazel.

Beck, A., Brown, G., Berchick, R., Stewart, B., & Steer, R. (1990). Relationship between hopelessness and ultimate suicide: A replication with psychiatric outpatients. *American Journal of Psychiatry, 147,* 190–195.

Beck, A., Rush, A., Shaw, B., & Emery, G. (1979). *Cognitive therapy of depression.* New York: Guilford.

Clarkin, J., Pilkonis, P., & Magrude, K. (1996). Psychotherapy of depression. *Archives of General Psychiatry, 53,* 717–723.

Coe, W. (1993). Expectations and hypnotherapy. In J. Rhue, S. Lynn, & I. Kirsch (Eds.), *Handbook of clinical hypnosis* (pp. 73–93). Washington, D.C.: American Psychological Association.

Cohen, D. (1994). *Out of the blue: Depression and human nature.* New York: Norton.

Cronkite, R., & Moos, R. (1995). Life context, coping processes, and depression. In E. Beckham and W. Leber (Eds.), *Handbook of depression* (pp. 569–587). New York: Guilford.

DeBattista, C., & Schatzberg, A. (1995). Somatic therapy. In I. Glick (Ed.), *Treating depression* (pp. 153–181). San Francisco: Jossey-Bass.

Depression Guideline Panel (1993). Clinical Practice Guideline Number 5: Depression in primary care. Volume 2: Treatment of Major Depression. Rockville, MD: U.S. Dept. of Health and Human Services, Agency for Health Care Policy and Research. AHCPR publication 93-0550.

Dubovsky, S. (1997). *Mind-body deceptions: The psychosomatics of everyday life.* New York: Norton.

Glass, R. (January 6, 1999). Treating depression as a recurrent or chronic disease. *Journal of the American Medical Association, 281,* 1, 83–84.

Greenberger, D., & Padesky, C. (1995). *Mind over mood.* New York: Guilford.

Haley, J. (1973). *Uncommon therapy: The uncommon psychiatric techniques of Milton H. Erickson, M.D.* New York: Norton.

Harvey, A. (2000). Pre-sleep cognitive activity: A comparison of sleep-onset insomniacs and good sleepers. *British Journal of Clinical Psychology, 39*(3), 275–286.

Hilgard, E. (1988). Personal communication.

Holahan, C., Moos, R., & Bonin, L. (1999). Social context and depression: An integrative stress and coping framework. In T. Joiner & J. Coyne (Eds.), *The interactional nature of depression* (pp. 39–63). Washington, D.C.: American Psychological Association.

Joiner, T., Coyne, J., & Blalock, J. (1999). On the interpersonal nature of depression: Overview and synthesis. In T. Joiner & J. Coyne (Eds.), *The interactional nature of depression: Advances in interpersonal approaches* (pp. 3–19). Washington, D.C.: American Psychological Association.

Just, N. & Alloy, L. (1997). The response styles theory of depression: Tests and an extension of the theory. _Journal of Abnormal Psychology, 106,_ 221–229.

Kaelber, C., Moul, D., & Farmer, M. (1995). Epidemiology of depression. In E. Beckham and W. Leber (Eds.), _Handbook of depression_ (pp. 3–35). New York: Guilford.

Kirsch, I. (1996). Hypnosis in psychotherapy: Efficacy and mechanisms. _Contemporary Hypnosis, 13_(2), 109–114.

Kirsch, I. (January/April, 2000). The response set theory of hypnosis. _American Journal of Clinical Hypnosis, 42,_ 3–4, 274–293.

Kirsch, I., Montgomery, G., & Sapirstein, G. (1995). Hypnosis as an adjunct to cognitive-behavioral psychotherapy: A meta-analysis. _Journal of Consulting and Clinical Psychology, 63,_ 214–220.

Lynn, S., & Kirsch, I. (2006). _Essentials of clinical hypnosis._ Washington, D.C.: American Psychological Association.

Lynn, S., Kirsch, I., Barabasz, A., Cardena, E., & Patterson, D. (April, 2000). Hypnosis as an empirically supported clinical intervention: The state of the evidence and a look to the future. _International Journal of Clinical and Experimental Hypnosis, 48_(2), 239–259.

Martell, C., Jacobson, N., & Addis, M. (2001). _Depression in context: Strategies for guided action._ New York: Norton.

Mondimore, F. (1993). _Depression: The mood disease._ Baltimore: Johns Hopkins University Press.

National Institute of Mental Health (NIMH). (2002). _Best estimate 1 year prevalence rates based on ECA and NCS, ages 18–54._ Bethesda, MD: Author.

Nolen-Hoeksema, S. (1991). Responses to depression and their effects on the duration of depressive episodes. _Journal of Abnormal Psychology, 100,_ 569–582.

Nolen-Hoeksema, S. (2000). The role of rumination in depressive disorder and mixed anxiety/depressive symptoms. _Journal of Abnormal Psychology, 109,_ 504–511.

Nolen-Hoeksema, S. (2003). _Women who think too much: How to break free of overthinking and reclaim your life._ New York: Henry Holt.

Peterson, C. (2000). The future of optimism. _American Psychologist, 55, 1,_ 44–55.

Phillips, M. (2006). Hypnosis with depression, posttraumatic stress disorder and chronic pain. In M. Yapko (Ed.), _Hypnosis and treating depression: Applications in clinical practice_ (pp. 217–241). New York: Brunner/Routledge.

Sarbin, T. (1997). Hypnosis as a conversation: "Believed-in imaginings" revisited. _Contemporary Hypnosis, 14, 4,_ 203–215.

Schoenberger, N. (April, 2000). Research on hypnosis as an adjunct to cognitive-behavioral psychotherapy. _International Journal of Clinical and Experimental Hypnosis, 48, 2,_ 154–169.

Schoenberger, N., Kirsch, I., Gearan, P., Montgomery, G., & Pastyrnak, S. (1997). Hypnotic enhancement of a cognitive behavioral treatment for public speaking anxiety. _Behavior Therapy, 28,_ 127–140.

Schulberg, H., Katon, W., Simon, G., & Rush, A. (December, 1998). Treating major depression in primary care practice. _Archives of General Psychiatry, 55,_ 1121–1127.

Schwartz, B. (2004). *The paradox of choice: Why more is less*. New York: Ecco.

Schwartz, J., & Begley, S. (2002). *The mind and the brain: Neuroplasticity and the power of mental force*. New York: HarperCollins.

Seligman, M. (1989). Explanatory style: Predicting depression, achievement, and health. In M. Yapko (Ed.), *Brief therapy approaches to treating anxiety and depression* (pp. 5–32). New York: Brunner/Mazel.

Seligman, M. (1990). *Learned optimism*. New York: Alfred A. Knopf.

Seligman, M. (2000). *American Psychologist: Special issue on happiness, excellence and optimal human functioning, 55 (1)*, 5–183.

Siever, L. (with Frucht, W.) (1997). *The new view of self*. New York: Macmillan.

Spasojevíc, J., & Alloy, L. (2001). Rumination as a common mechanism relating depressive risk factors to depression. *Emotion, 1*, 25–37.

Stevens, D., Merikangas, K., & Merikangas, J. (1995). Comorbidity of depression and other medical conditions. In E. Beckham and W. Leber (Eds.), *Handbook of depression* (pp. 147–199). New York: Guilford.

Thase, M. (2000). Treatment issues related to sleep and depression. *Journal of Clinical Psychiatry, 61* (suppl. 11), 46–50.

Thase, M., & Glick, I. (1995). Combined treatment. In I. Glick (Ed.), *Treating depression* (pp. 183–208). San Francisco: Jossey-Bass.

Thase, M., & Howland, R. (1995). Biological processes in depression: An updated review and integration. In E. Beckham & W. Leber (Eds.), *Handbook of depression* (pp. 213–279). New York: Guilford.

Torem, M. (1987). Hypnosis in the treatment of depression. In W. Wester (Ed.), *Clinical hypnosis: A case management approach* (p. 288–301). Cincinnati, OH: Behavioral Science Center.

Torem, M. (1992). Back from the future: A powerful age progression technique. *American Journal of Clinical Hypnosis, 35*(2), 81–88.

Torem, M. (2006). Treating depression: A remedy from the future. In M. Yapko (Ed.), *Hypnosis and treating depression: Applications in clinical practice* (pp. 97–119). New York: Brunner/Routledge.

Weissbourd, R. (1996). *The vulnerable child: What really hurts America's children and what we can do about it*. Reading, PA: Addison-Wesley.

Yapko, M. (1988). *When living hurts: Directives for treating depression*. New York: Brunner/Mazel.

Yapko, M. (1992). *Hypnosis and the treatment of depressions*. New York: Brunner/Mazel.

Yapko, M. (1993). Hypnosis and depression. In J. Rhue, S. Lynn & I. Kirsch (Eds.), *Handbook of clinical hypnosis* (pp. 339–355). Washington, D.C.: American Psychological Association.

Yapko, M. (1997). *Breaking the patterns of depression*. New York: Random House/Doubleday.

Yapko, M. (1999). *Hand-me-down blues: How to stop depression from spreading in families*. New York: St. Martin's Griffin.

Yapko, M. (2001). *Treating depression with hypnosis: Integrating cognitive-behavioral and strategic approaches*. Philadelphia, PA: Brunner/Routledge.

Yapko, M. (2003). *Trancework: An introduction to the practice of clinical hypnosis* (3rd ed.). New York: Brunner/Routledge.

Yapko, M. (Ed.) (2006). *Hypnosis and treating depression: Applications in clinical practice.* New York: Brunner/Routledge.

Zeig, J. (Ed.) (1980). *A teaching seminar with Milton H. Erickson, M.D.* New York: Brunner/Mazel.

Chapter 5

Hypnosis in Interventional Radiology and Outpatient Procedure Settings

Nicole Flory and Elvira Lang

OVERVIEW

Over the past decades, surgery has evolved from the traditional large-incision technique to minimally invasive approaches, fueled by a revolution in medical imaging and device design. Skilled specialists can now insert surgical instruments through tiny skin openings under the guidance of X-rays, ultrasound, magnet resonance imaging (MRI), or endoscopes. The field of interventional radiology has blossomed from these advancements, and other specialties have adopted the minimally invasive approaches pioneered in radiology. Many surgeries that previously required general anesthesia and prolonged hospital stays are now outpatient procedures. While patients greatly benefit from these developments, high-tech procedures still involve considerable physical and psychological risks for patients who can now remain alert and conscious on the operating table. In addition, indications for interventions have expanded to include more fragile patients, who in the past would have been excluded from more traditional treatment, and these patients require an even greater degree of care.

Managing procedural distress in the interventional radiology suite and other outpatient procedure settings remains a challenge for clinicians and patients. Treatment teams typically rely on local anesthetics and drugs to counteract pain and anxiety. Although generally safe, these can have limited effectiveness and serious side effects. With the public's increasing interest in more holistic approaches, that is, a combination of high tech and high touch, and mounting scientific evidence for alterative approaches, use of hypnosis in the procedural setting shows great promise. This chapter will touch on the specifics of the setting, and the premise, attractiveness and challenges of using hypnosis during surgery in conscious patients.

HYPNOSIS IN THE EVOLUTION OF SURGICAL AND ANESTHETIC APPROACHES

In the evolution of surgery, development of instrumentation, anesthesia, and infection-free healing have been intimately intertwined. Progress in one of these domains fuels progress in the others, and conversely, without progress of all three, the field cannot progress effectively. In the nineteenth century, the Scottish surgeon James Esdaile started to use hypnotic techniques in India mainly out of desperation for lack of other means of pain control (Esdaile, 1946/1957). He had heard of Franz Mesmer in Vienna who had gained fame curing mainly psychosomatic illnesses through hypnotic and trance-like states. Esdaile had never seen a "mesmeric" session, but read about its use for medical procedures. He successfully used these techniques during major surgery. He not only found that patients experienced less pain, but also noticed that the rate of infection was greatly reduced. However, with the discovery of the clinical use of ether and shortly thereafter chloroform, clinicians gave preference to the use of pharmaceuticals for pain control and the initial excitement about hypnosis in the operating room diminished. In 1846, Morton first gave ether to patients for dental procedures and then demonstrated its use to the public in an amphitheater later known as "Ether Dome" at the Massachusetts General Hospital (Skolnick, 1996). In 1847, Simpson first used chloroform on women during child birth (Simpson, 1847), which caused much controversy and contempt among certain religious groups (Mander, 1998). The initial enthusiasm for ether and chloroform, however, was damped by serious side effects and deaths following surgery (Duffy, 1964). This was mainly due to poor safety considerations, over sedation, and the spread of infection—in particular, during labor and delivery involving physicians (Mander, 1998). In 1847, Semmelweiss contributed a milestone to the evolution of surgery (Grant, Grant, & Lockwood, 2005). By promoting hand washing with 4 percent chlorinated lime solution for doctors and their trainees assisting in childbirth, he was able to reduce maternal mortality from 13–30 percent to 1.2 percent (Nuland, 2003). Thus, he brought about one of the most important steps in reducing wound infection and mortality. Unfortunately, Semmelweis's efforts were met with much hostility and hand washing was accepted only years later, after his death, as a principle of antisepsis in surgery (Grant et al., 2005). His experience may serve as an example that simple measures with obvious positive patient outcomes still can face great opposition from members of the medical community who adhere to ingrained but unproven customs.

With the progress made in the nineteenth century, surgeons of the twentieth century were ready to expand to an extensive array of open surgeries including large abdominal incisions and chest operations with heart lung machines. In the last decades, technical evolution has permitted less-invasive methods to address the same "plumbing needs" with speedier recovery. Specially trained physicians can now insert miniature high-tech devices through the patient's skin under the guidance of various imaging techniques. These imaging techniques include X-rays, ultrasound, computer tomography, MRI, or endoscopes. For example, pus, kidney stones, gall bladders, and tumors can now be removed without cutting patients open. Interventionalists can now open blocked arteries, veins, or bile ducts from the inside through image-guided surgical interventions. The new subspecialty of radiology, called interventional radiology, and subsequently, interventional pulmonary, gastroenterology, cardiology, vascular, and general surgery have all profited tremendously from advances in minimally invasive surgery.

In conjunction with the evolution of surgical techniques, the modes of chemical anesthesia have also expanded. Local anesthetics with varying times of actions have been devised, and drugs that counteract pain and anxiety are continuously evolving. For minimally invasive surgery, general anesthesia is no longer necessary. Interventionalists usually administer injections of local anesthetic medication (such as lidocaine) in conjunction with analgesic agents and intravenous (IV) "conscious" or "moderate sedation" (Lang, Chen, Fick, & Berbaum, 1998; Martin & Lennox, 2003). While these drug regimens generally are well tolerated during procedures, they are not always effective and can have side effects including cardiovascular problems, cessation of breathing (apnea), shortage of oxygen (hypoxia), unconsciousness (coma), and very rarely death (Martin & Lennox, 2003).

While serious complications during minimally invasive procedures are rare, even a very low incidence of adverse events has larger-scale consequences. For example, millions of routine endoscopies are performed. Experts estimate that 3–13 percent of patients will face complications or other adverse outcome following their endoscopy (Mahnke et al., 2006). About 750 per 100,000 individuals undergo endoscopies for upper gastrointestinal problems annually (British National Institute for Health and Clinical Excellence; Web page 12/11/2006). In the United States, experts suspect that endoscopies result in more than 70,000 serious complications each year. Therefore, any medical intervention should be used judiciously to provide the best care to patients (Martin, Lennox, & Buckley, 2005).

The occurrence of adverse effects not only depends on the type of procedure performed, but also on the amount and properties of each medication as well as the patient's susceptibility to certain medical problems (Hatsiopoulou, Cohen, & Lang, 2003). Research findings document that the amount of medication for the same medical procedure differs significantly between patients, health care providers, and hospital settings (Gracely, McGrath, Heft, & Dubner, 1977; Lang et al., 1998). The risk associated with the use of monitored anesthesia during minimally invasive procedures can be comparable to that seen in general anesthesia. It is thus not surprising to see a rekindling of interest in hypnosis for the management of procedural distress.

In the nineteenth century, the development of pharmacologic anesthesia greatly reduced the use of hypnosis during surgery (D. Spiegel, 2006; Wain, 2004), but a small group of dedicated physicians continued using hypnotic techniques solely or as an adjunct throughout the century. Hypnosis was then mainly used for individuals who had a contraindication to chemical anesthesia or purposefully requested a hypnotic intervention (Blankfield, 1991). While use of general anesthesia permitted development of extensive open surgery, it also opened the way to minimally invasive techniques that now no longer require general anesthesia. In the twenty-first century, we may well have reached the point where the greatest procedural risks are those related to the patients' pain, anxiety, and the management of these symptoms. Greater requests for transparency in medicine and the requirements of hospitals to share complication rates with the public make non-pharmacologic methods, with their high safety profile and the potential for high patient satisfaction, once again a very attractive alternative.

PROCEDURAL ENVIRONMENT

Despite the "minimally invasive" label, procedures in interventional radiology or other outpatient settings are not free of pain and possible distress. During outpatient surgery or minimally invasive procedures, patients typically remain conscious and immobilized on a table, sometimes for several hours, and in cases where image guidance is necessary, the room is darkened to permit viewing of the monitors. Instruments such as wires, catheters, and endoscopes that can measure several feet in length are inserted into various openings. If one were to design a psychological experiment to create feelings of anxiety and despair, one would likely choose most of the elements present in the procedure room: fear for life or health, loss of control, uncertainty of outcome, presence of masked strangers, darkness, immobilization, exposure and vulnerability (Flory, Salazar, & Lang, 2007).

Even for generally healthy and well-adjusted individuals, a visit to the operating room can be a stressful experience. Patients often experience worry and concern, such as fear about being in pain, giving up control, loss of body image or physical attractiveness, surgical complications, adverse reactions to anesthesia, and death (Anderson & Masur, 1983). Optimal patient care involving heavy reliance on technology-based interventions like radiology procedures should expand to include much needed emotional support for patients (Peteet et al., 1992). Reducing anticipatory anxiety is not only desirable in itself but also has considerable implications for the upcoming procedure. In a study with patients undergoing interventional radiological procedures, pre-procedure anxiety significantly correlated with anxiety, pain, and medication use and overall procedure length (Schupp,

Berbaum, Berbaum, & Lang, 2005). Highly anxious patients ask for and are offered more medication during surgery, therefore exposing them to a greater likelihood of adverse events. Pain and distress can also result in a longer stay in the recovery room, additional medication use, delayed discharge, and hospital readmission (Chung, Ritchie, & Su, 1997). Recovery from surgery is of vital importance since all the mentioned adverse events put additional strain on the patients and at the same time inflate health care costs (Montgomery et al., 2007).

BASES OF PROCEDURAL PAIN MANAGEMENT WITH HYPNOSIS

The experience of pain is a complex and highly subjective phenomenon (Price, Harkins, & Baker, 1987). The same physical stimuli that may be barely noticed as painful could be experienced as excruciating in a different setting, or as David Spiegel once described the phenomenon, "the strain in the pain is in the brain." Focused attention and awareness are key elements in changing perceptions of pain (Spiegel & Spiegel, 1978). For example, intense attention toward an imagined warm and tingling sensation may modify the brain's response to the painful signal (Spiegel & Bloom, 1983). Pain is usually perceived in different dimensions according to its sensory, cognitive, and affective-emotional aspects (Melzack, 1999). Hypnosis can reduce both the sensory and affective dimensions of pain, thereby reducing overall pain perception (Wright & Drummond, 2000). Magnetic resonance imaging studies have demonstrated that the wording of hypnotic suggestions can systematically alter the brain's processing of the same painful stimulus. Suggestions targeting the sensory dimensions of pain resulted in a modulation of activity in the primary sensatory cortex, while suggestions targeting the affective components of pain resulted in changes in the anterior cingulated cortex (Rainville, Bao, & Chretien, 2005; Rainville, Carrier, Hofbauer, Bushnell, & Duncan, 1999; Rainville, Duncan, Price, Carrier, & Bushnell, 1997). Pain and anxiety are interrelated (Schupp et al., 2005), and reduction of one is likely to beneficially affect the other.

Hypnotic techniques can be considered brief therapeutic interventions changing cognitions, emotions, and behaviors of individuals. Hypnotic analgesia lets patients explore their own capacity to interact with a painful or uncomfortable situation (Spiegel et al., 1989). Its benefits have been documented for patients in various settings with no or little side effects (Faymonville et al., 1995; Huth, Broome, & Good, 2004; Lang et al., 2000). This is in contradiction to the purely pharmacologic approach. While pharmacologic treatments for pain and anxiety may seem like a quick fix, clinical experience shows that the adrenergic activation of very anxious patients can override even large amounts of sedatives and narcotics. This adrenergic activation does not only render chemical drugs ineffective, but is also dangerous once the procedure is over and the full drug effect suddenly emerges. In this context it seems much more efficient to engage in a quick hypnotic anxiety conversion up front. On the other hand, one should not be opposed to judicious use of drugs or place performance pressure on patients and their hypnosis providers. It is important to offer patients the choice of hypnosis, drugs, both, or none in what they perceive as their needs within the realm of safety. Earlier concerns of some, that sedatives and analgesics may adversely affect a patient's ability to engage with hypnosis on the procedure table, have not been proven in a series of clinical studies. These have shown that procedural pain and anxiety can be well managed through a combination of relatively small amounts of medication and hypnosis in a wide range of medical procedures (Baglini et al., 2004; Butler, Symons, Henderson, Shortliffe, & Spiegel, 2005; Lang et al., 2000; Lang et al., 2006; Stewart, 2005).

HYPNOTIC TECHNIQUES

Since this book describes hypnotic techniques and general principles, we will explain approaches that are more specific to interventional radiology and other outpatient medical settings. The interventional procedure suite can be noisy, sabotage prone, and buzzing with different activities. This environment is very different from the practice of a therapist or psychologist with a couch in a tranquil office setting. While an office setting allows 40-minute inductions, the generation of patient-specific tapes, and possibly subsequent patient practice at home, the procedure environment requires quick action.

In the ideal case, hypnosis in the procedure room should be provided by a person who is already part of the team (Blankfield, 1991). This person would have had the opportunity to meet the patient on a prior visit and used the opportunity to learn the patient's individual responses to stressful situations. In our experience this is highly unlikely in the current cost- and time-conscious culture of medicine. Often, the needs and provisions for each individual patient can only be established once the patient has arrived in the procedure room. Rapid attention to such needs and brief interventions are essential. Emphasis should be placed on building rapid rapport, positive wording of suggestions, openness to discussion, and use of patient-centered imagery. On the other hand, patients are highly suggestible in the health care setting and, in particular, the acute care area (H. Spiegel, 1997), so that lengthy inductions are not necessary. Also, the approach should not interfere with patient preparation for the surgery and surgery itself. Although hypnosis is still highly cost effective even if it adds procedure time (Lang & Rosen, 2002; Montgomery et al., 2007), it has been very difficult in our experience to convey to procedure personnel that halting their activity—even for a little while and contrary to the evidence—could bring any good at all. We have learned over the years that it is very well possible to start the hypnotic process while a patient is being "prepped" (e.g., cleansed with antimicrobial solution), hooked up to equipment, or even when being positioned in a mammography unit.

To guide patients into self-hypnotic relaxation, we typically use scripts; yet these are structured such that flexibility, openness, and patient-centered imagery are all key elements. The overpowering aspect of technology in the procedure room is well offset by a highly permissive, responsive, and interactive approach that conveys a greater sense of control for the patient (Flory et al., 2007). It therefore mirrors some of the key aspects of Ericksonian hypnosis. Some argue that a deeper explorative non-scripted approach could produce even better results (Barabasz & Christensen, 2006), but such requires very highly skilled hypnotists, which typically are not available on a daily basis in the clinical setting.

Seeing a hypnosis provider sit down to read a script can reduce misperceptions of hypnosis, overcome resistance, and provide comfort for both patients and health care professionals. A script can be a safety blanket that conveys how important the wording is when the patient lies on the operating table. It permits the whole treatment team to learn and reinforce hypnotic vocabulary. In addition, the use of scripts enables a greater standardization of treatment that is essential for documentation and reproducibility. It also permits the exchange of personnel during procedures and allows patients to drift in and out of hypnosis as they wish.

All hypnosis should be considered self-hypnosis as patients explore their own abilities to deal with painful or distressing stimuli. A semantic shift from "hypnosis" to "self-hypnosis" emphasizes the patient's active participation. Patients often feel out of control, passive, exposed, and vulnerable. Imagery that patients used to describe this state ranged from a "piece of red meat with a butcher knife all the way through," to "a little mouse being chase by huge barn cats," or "surrounded by knights in silver armors ready to pierce me." In the same way that these patients can produce distressing imagery, they can also envision more resourceful scenarios if guided appropriately. It is best to teach patients to help themselves, and patients take pride and fulfillment in being able to produce such scenarios. Their choices are highly individual—another reason why we do not believe "one-size-fits-all" hypnosis tapes. What pleases some patients may be disturbing to others as in the following examples: camping on the Mississippi, floating on the clouds with one's deceased relatives, flying a plane in the dark night sky, gambling in Las Vegas, or even canning vegetables while watching TV (Fick, Lang, Benotsch, Lutgendorf, & Logan, 1999).

There are many ways to structure the hypnotic process in the procedure room; based on our experience, we describe what we found most useful in our setting. The approach contains two elements. The first is a set of structured attentive behaviors that the hypnosis provider displays in the first seconds of the patient encounter. The second element is the reading of the script in the next section.

We have reported that hypnosis in the operating room should also include other techniques in addition to hypnosis such as structured attentive behaviors, establishing rapport, correct use of language and suggestions, patient-initiated imagery, relaxation training, and provisions to address patients' worries as early as possible (Lang et al., 1999). Structured attentive behavior consists of several behaviors, most importantly listening. Attentive listening is the key to instant rapport building—the listener seeks to understand and uses patient-generated images for the hypnosis. A second element is matching the patients' verbal and nonverbal behavior pattern; examples include sitting at eye level with the patient and the removal of barriers between the patient and the hypnosis provider in the operating room. Other elements of attentive behaviors include provision for increasing the patient's perception of control by prompt responses to patient requests. Last, but not least, encouragement presented in statements like "thank you for your cooperation" will empower the patient to take a more active role during his or her medical treatment (Lang et al., 1999).

The correct use of language and suggestions is important since patients generally present to the operating room with heightened suggestibility (H. Spiegel, 1997). Negatively loaded suggestions such has "sharp pain and pressure now" or "this will hurt a bit" can reinforce anxiety and magnify attention to pain (Lang et al., 2005). Emotionally neutral descriptions are preferable and may include "feeling of warmth and fullness" or "focus on the sensation of your breath." Positive suggestions foster relaxation, and patient-centered imagery around successful coping will enhance the patient's well-being (Erickson, 1994). It is best to tap into the already existing coping strategies by using the patient's words and descriptions.

SCRIPT

There are many options for hypnosis scripts. After having worked with several scripts and learned from our pitfalls, Dr. D. Spiegel helped us develop the following script, which was tested for efficacy in several randomized-controlled trials (Lang et al., 1999; Lang et al., 2006). Over the years we made small changes based on feedback from the hypnosis community. For individuals who wish to develop their own scripts, we recommend that the following elements be included: a short explanation about what is going to happen, use of an induction that can be repeated should other personnel or events sabotage the process and inadvertently re-alert the patient, an immunization against the noise and interruptions in the room as well as unhelpful suggestions, a simple way to engage in resourceful imagery, elements of anxiety and pain conversion if needed, and a reorientation that acknowledges the patient's contribution.

"We want you to help us to help you to learn a concentration exercise to help you get through the procedure more comfortably. It can be a way to help your body be more comfortable through the procedure and also deal with any discomfort that may come up during the procedure. It is just a form of concentration, like getting so caught up in a movie or a good book that you forget you are watching a movie or reading a book.

Now you may be interested to learn how you can use your imagination to enter a state of focused attention and physical relaxation. If you hear sounds or noises in the room, just use these to deepen your experience. And use only the suggestions that are helpful for you. There are a lot of ways to relax, but here is one simple way:

On one, you can do one thing—look up.
On two, two things, slowly close your eyes and take a deep breath.
On three, three things, breath out, relax your eyes, and let your body float.

That's good, just imagine your whole body floating, floating through the table, each breath deeper and easier. Right now you might imagine that you are floating somewhere safe and comfortable, in a bath, a lake, a hot tub, or just floating in space, each breath deeper and easier. Just notice how with each breath you let a little more tension out of your body as you let your whole body float, safe and comfortable, each breath deeper and easier. Good, now with your eyes closed and remaining in this state of concentration, please describe for me how your body is feeling right now. Where do you imagine yourself being? What is it like? Can you smell the air? Can you see what is around you? Good, now this is your safe and pleasant place to be and you can use it in a sense to play a trick on the doctors. Your body has to be here, but you don't. So just spend your time being somewhere you would rather be.

Now, if there is some discomfort, and there may be some with the procedure as they prepare you and insert the line, or as you feel the dye entering your body, there is no point in fighting it. You can admit it, but then transform that sensation. If you feel some discomfort, you might find it helpful to make that part of your body to feel warmer, as if you were in a bath. Or cooler, if that is more comfortable, as if you had ice or snow on that part of your body. This warmth and coolness becomes a protective filter between you and the pain.

If you have any discomfort right now imagine that you are applying a hot pack or you are putting snow or ice on it and see what it feels like. Develop the sense of warm or cool tingling numbness to filter the hurt out of the pain.

With each breath, breathe deeper and easier, your body is floating, filter the hurt out of the pain.

Now again with your eyes closed and remaining in the state of concentration, describe what you are feeling right now.

(1) *If they are at their safe and comfortable place—reinforce it.*
What is it like now? What do you see around you? What are you doing?

(2) *If they are in pain*—The pain is there but see if you can add coolness, more warmth, or make it lighter or heavier.

If no longer in pain—Good, continue to focus on those sensations.

If still in pain—Try to focus on sensations in another part of your body. Now rub your fingertips together and notice all of the delicate sensations in your fingertips and see how much you can observe about what it feels like to rub your thumb and forefingers together. How do you feel now?

If not in pain—Good, continue to focus on these sensations.

If still in pain—Now imagine yourself being at _____ (patient's safe place) where you said you felt relaxed and comfortable. What is it like now? What is the temperature? What do you see around you?

(3) *If they state that they are worried*—Okay, your main job right now is to help your body feel comfortable, so we will talk about what is worrying you. But first, no matter what we discuss, concentrate on your body floating. So let's get the floating back into your body. Imagine that you are in this favorite spot and when you are ready let me know by nodding your head and then we will talk about what is worrying you. But remember no matter what we discuss concentrate on your body floating, and feel safe and comfortable. So what is worrying you? (*Discuss*)

How do you feel now? *If not worried*: Good, now continue to concentrate on body floating, and feel safe and comfortable in your favorite place.

If after discussing patient has persistent worry, then—Okay you might picture in your mind a screen like a movie screen, TV screen, or a piece of clear blue sky. First you might see a pleasant scene on it. Now you may picture a large piece of blue screen divided in half. All right, now on the left half, picture what you are worrying about on the screen. Now on the right half, picture what you will do about it, or what you would recommend someone else to do about it. Keep your body floating, and if you are worrying about the outcome, okay admit it to yourself, but your body does not have to get uptight about it. You may, but your body does not have to. Good, you know that whatever happens there is always something you can do. But for now just concentrate on keeping your body floating and feeling safe and comfortable.

Sometimes throughout the procedure say—If you feel any sense of discomfort you are welcome to let me know about it. You may use the filter to filter the hurt out of the pain, but by all means let me know and I will do what I can to help you with it as well. Whatever you do just keep your body floating and concentrate on being in the place where you feel safe and comfortable.

When finished, say—Okay the procedure is over now. We are going to leave formally this state of concentration by counting backwards from three to one. On three get ready, on two with your eyes closed roll up your eyes, and on one let your eyes open and take a deep breath and let it out.

That will be the end of the formal exercise, but when you come out of it you will still have the feeling of comfort that you felt during it. Ready, three, two, one.

If necessary: Three—get ready. Two—with your eyes closed roll up your eyes. One—let your eyes open and take a deep breath, and feel refreshed and proud about having helped yourself through this procedure."

SCIENTIFIC EVIDENCE

For the past century, the majority of research on hypnosis has been in the form of case reports, often based on the descriptions of the treating clinician. Supporters of evidence-based medicine often frown on the lack of thorough methodology; for example, use of anecdotal case reports, selection biases, retrospective designs, non-standardized interventions, or vague outcome measures. As such, hypnosis had suffered from lack of availability of such data from randomized studies (Blankfield, 1991). Nowadays, however, empirical support for the effectiveness of hypnotic techniques for medical purposes is available from both experimental and clinical studies. Modern developments in neuro-imaging provide insight into the physiological mechanism of hypnosis. In experimental studies, hypnotic instructions have been shown to alter the way pain or other distressful events are processed in the brain and perceived by an individual (Rainville et al., 2005; Rainville et al., 1999; Rainville et al., 1997). For example, changing the wording of suggestions under hypnosis affects the activation of different brain centers during exposure to the same stimulus (Rainville et al., 1997). Rainville et al. (1997) demonstrated that suggestions targeting the sensory dimension of the pain (such as "you will feel a tingling sensation") resulted in activation changes in the primary sensory cortex. Suggestions targeting the affective dimension of the pain (such as "you will remain calm") resulted in changes in the anterior cingulate cortex.

Clinical studies with superior methodology using prospective randomized control designs have demonstrated the effectiveness of hypnotic techniques in the peri-operative domain, that is, before (Saadat & Kain, 2007), during (Lang et al., 2000; Lang et al., 2006), and after surgery (Huth et al., 2004). To name a few examples, hypnotic techniques have been used for various treatment of breast cancer, burn care, plastic surgery, tumor embolization, labor and delivery, and the removal of appendices, bone marrow, teeth, and tonsils (Butler et al., 2005; Faymonville et al., 1995; Huth et al., 2004; Lang et al., 2000; Lang et al., 2006; Montgomery et al., 2007; Patterson, Questad, & deLateour, 1989; Wright & Drummond, 2000; Zeltzer & LeBaron, 1982).

Faymonville et al. (2000) reviewed 1,650 various surgical procedures from retrospective and randomized prospective studies in which hypnosis was used as an adjunctive treatment to conscious sedation. The authors concluded that patients greatly benefited from hypnosis as a result of greater active participation, procedural comfort, faster recovery time, and shorter hospital stays. To date, the literature on hypnosis documents that this brief psychological intervention significantly reduces pain intensity, pain unpleasantness, anxiety, nausea, fatigue, medication use, and procedure time (Butler et al., 2005; Faymonville et al., 2000; Lang et al., 2000; Lang et al., 2005; Montgomery et al., 2007).

Montgomery, David, Winkel, Silverstein, & Bovberg (2002) conducted a meta-analysis of 20 randomized-controlled trials evaluating the effectiveness of hypnotic techniques in conjunction with pharmacologic treatments for various medical procedures. Results indicated that on average about 90 percent of surgical patients profited from adjunctive treatment compared to control groups. Outcomes were evaluated according to negative affect, pain, medication, recovery, and treatment time; hypnosis produced better results in all of these domains. The authors concluded that hypnosis is an effective adjunctive procedure for a wide variety of surgical patients (Montgomery et al., 2002).

Particularly in the realm of interventional radiology, using interventions with documented beneficial outcomes that are safe and easy to apply on the procedure table is of prime concern. The current gold standard to assess efficacy and treatment safety is evidence from prospective randomized controlled trials in which patients are randomly assigned to different treatment conditions. In the experimental group, patients receive an intervention such as a self-hypnotic relaxation exercise. In the control group, patients receive the standard medical care without any specific intervention or without an additional person attending to them. There is an ongoing debate as to which group of patients represents an appropriate control group. Jensen and Patterson (2005) have argued that an additional control should be included that does not receive hypnosis or pharmacologic treatment. However, the intervention still needs to be credible but minimally effective to control for the social aspects and additional care through the hypnosis provider present in the hypnosis condition (Jensen & Patterson, 2005).

Lang et al. (2000) presented the most comprehensive study using a prospective randomized-controlled design to establish hypnosis outcomes to date. In this study, 241 patients underwent interventional radiology procedures in the kidneys and vascular system. Patients were randomized to self-hypnotic relaxation, structured attention, and standard care. All patients had access to local anesthetic and IV medication if they requested it. Hypnosis significantly reduced anxiety, pain, drug use, and complications. As a result, procedure time was reduced by 17 minutes compared to standard care. In addition, hypnosis reduced costs an average of $330 per procedure compared to standard care (Lang & Rosen, 2002).

Lang et al. (2006) conducted another randomized-controlled trial on 236 women undergoing large core breast biopsies comparing hypnosis to standard care and empathic attention. Large core breast biopsies are known to often cause distress in patients and are usually performed solely under a local anesthesia (Bugbee et al., 2005). Hypnosis and empathic attention were administered in addition to local anesthesia; both significantly reduced pain perception, but only hypnosis also reduced anxiety (Lang et al., 2006).

Montgomery et al. (2007) have presented the most recent randomized study on brief hypnosis interventions in 200 patients undergoing breast cancer surgery. Women were randomized to either a pre-operative hypnosis session with a psychologist or non-directive empathic listening (attention control). Hypnosis resulted in significantly less drug use for sedation and pain management during the procedure compared to the control group. Patients in the hypnosis group also reported less pain, nausea, fatigue, discomfort, and emotional upset than the controls. The authors also documented that hypnosis reduced costs by $772.71 per patient for the institution, mainly as a result of shorter stays in the procedure room (Montgomery et al., 2007).

In summary, there is overwhelming support for the effectiveness of hypnosis to manage pain and anxiety in patients undergoing invasive medical procedures. In addition, complications and cost can be reduced by its use.

PATIENTS RESPONSIVENESS AND ACCEPTANCE

In recent years, patients have become more educated about their health and surgical interventions. Patients want to become more actively involved in their care. This includes using alternative treatments to reduce pain and distress. Western medicine has traditionally not met these needs, and patients have therefore turned toward more alternative sources of healing. About a third of Americans use alternative treatments for their medical problems, and it is therefore not surprising that patients present with their own coping strategies to the procedure suite (Campion, 1993; Eisenberg et al., 1993). Many patients use mind-body techniques that can reduce pain and anxiety including imagery, distraction, relaxation, hypnosis, and meditation (Quirk, Letenre, Ciottone, & Lingley, 1989; Astin, 2004; Astin, Shapiro, Eisenberg, & Forys, 2003).

In recent years, the Internet, books, and tapes have become valuable tools for patients, and their authors claim extensive widespread use. It is becoming more common to see patients checking in for their procedures with hypnosis tapes or requests for specific coping rituals. Introduction of hypnosis into the procedure suite may thus become a consumer-driven event. As David Spiegel (2007) recently stated, hypnotic techniques suffered the "disadvantage" of not involving drugs or other products that can be purchased. If this were the case, the industry would have worked hard to try selling this product. However, the tide may be turning in favor of such patient-centered therapy based on patient demand and the superior outcome profile for procedures performed under hypnosis. What held true for Esdaile in the nineteenth century still holds in the twenty-first century—hospitals with better outcomes will attract more patients, and healthcare facilities would be advised to take note in order to compete in the consumer-driven market of health care.

The question then becomes, which patients can benefit from hypnosis during surgery? Highly hypnotizable individuals have undergone open surgery solely under hypnosis without general or local anesthesia (Wain, 2004). Wain (2004) has described these talented patients as "hypnotic virtuosos," but these represent only a small percentage of patients. However, even hypnosis-naive and moderately hypnotizable individuals can be guided quickly into self-hypnotic relaxation during minimally invasive procedures as described previously. For minimally invasive surgery that does not require general anesthesia, patients can benefit from hypnosis even when their hypnotizability is average or low (Flick et al., 1999). A recent study showed that in a cohort of patients aged 18–92, age had no effect on hypnotizability (Lutgendorf et al., 2007), a finding contradictory to previous reports (Morgan & Hilgard, 1972).

CHALLENGES

Despite the empirical support for the effectiveness of hypnotic techniques, hypnosis is still underused. Reasons for the slow acceptance of hypnosis into mainstream medicine are numerous and include inaccurate perceptions of this practice. One such inaccurate perception is that hypnosis requires additional time and financial costs (Anbar, 2006); the opposite has been documented (Lang & Rosen, 2002; Montgomery et al., 2007). Another reason for slow acceptance may rest with the fact that successful use of hypnosis in the procedure room depends on the cooperation of all members of the treatment team. Treatments that depend on interpersonal skills and not a technical gadget are often met with skepticism and sometimes ridiculed by more empirically trained health care professionals.

Research findings on the effectiveness of audio tapes and computerized interventions have been mixed (Ghoneim, Block, Sarasin, Davis, & Marchman, 2000; Hart, 1980). It appears that such interventions can be effective for both treatment outcomes and costs, but more patient-centered approaches with a personal hypnosis provider have resulted in more consistent benefits. As attractive as it might be to give patients a tape or some high-tech device such as virtual reality helmets developed by Patterson et al. (2006), proceedings in the operating room are complex. Providing patients with the best medical care including procedural hypnosis requires that the patient's individual preferences are respected and that the whole treatment team is willing to go along or at least not to interfere. It "takes a village" to attend to the patient's needs and solicit the collaboration of everybody in the procedural suite for a successful outcome.

Some medical providers believe that stating how painful and distressing a procedure can be helps the patient and expresses sympathy. With good intentions physicians and nurses often use terms with unpleasant content such as "stinging sensation," "is it hurting yet," "don't worry, it will be over soon," or "sharp burning pain." It is assumed that such words help patients, but the opposite has been shown to be true (Lang et al., 2005). Such negatively loaded suggestions can create "nocebo effects" and increase pain and anxiety (H. Spiegel, 1997). The idea that words can both heal or harm is far from new. One of the oldest documents on medical practice, the "Hippocratic Corpus," explicitly states that physicians should pay attention to both talk and silence (Jones, 1923/1972).

Compassionate and empathic communication is often considered essential for good medical practice and has become an important part in training health care professionals. However, there remains considerable debate around what constitutes real empathy and whether it improves the patient's well-being. A recent study by Lang et al. (unpublished manuscript) found that hypnosis techniques and empathic attention reduce pain, anxiety, and medication during interventional radiology procedures. Yet, empathic techniques alone, without tapping into the patient's self-coping, resulted in more pain, anxiety, and complications. These complications were related not only to psychosocial well-being but also to adverse effects on blood pressure and oxygen supply. Just providing emotional support without guiding the patient into a more relaxed state seems counterproductive. Chatting and touching the patient may not only be unhelpful, but potentially harmful if not practiced with caution. Trying to be nice does not suffice in helping patients help themselves.

PRECAUTIONS AND SAFETY CONSIDERATIONS

Safety of the patient needs to be considered first before any procedures are implemented. Research studies on the medical use of hypnosis suggest that it carries little risk for adverse effects, and patients are generally satisfied with outcomes (Jensen et al., 2006). If adverse effects emerge, these are usually minor and transient. Possible adverse effects of hypnosis in the experimental context include drowsiness and headaches (Coe & Ryken, 1979). Therefore, several safety precautions should be considered and the potential for adverse effects needs to be recognized early (Barber, 1998).

Since comprehensive training in hypnosis is associated with a lesser likelihood of adverse effects (Lynn, Martin, & Frauman, 1996) its practice should be limited to health care professionals with adequate training. Health care professional should use hypnosis as an adjunct for a treatment that they are trained to deliver in the first place. For example, members of the treatment team in the interventional radiology suite could deliver hypnosis in the procedure room but should not attempt to treat post-traumatic stress syndrome. Hypnotic techniques should also not be used as the only tool or the last resort to manage pain, anxiety, or medical emergencies. As a precaution, it is not recommended that hypnosis be used with patients whose reality testing is compromised since mental health professionals are best qualified to treat this population. However, psychotic patients typically are not very hypnotizable (D. Spiegel, Detrick, & Frischolz, 1982).

Lang and colleagues have shown that hypnotic techniques are safe and effective in the interventional radiology setting (Lang, Joyce, Spiegel, Hamilton, & Lee, 1996). Use of hypnotic scripts can ensure safety and reproducibility that are particularly important in research and procedural settings. The script used by our group places an emphasis on rapid trance induction, patient-centered imagery, and permissiveness, and was originally developed by Dr. D. Spiegel (Lang et al., 1999). The script is quick and easy to apply, immune to disruptions, and also addresses fears of patients early before these become more difficult to manage.

CONCLUSIONS

Research has demonstrated that hypnotic techniques can be safely and effectively integrated into a medical high-tech environment. Integration of hypnosis in modern medicine does not add costs nor time. Even hypnosis-naive patients can learn hypnotic techniques on the operating table without disturbing or prolonging the procedure. In summary, hypnosis is ideally suited as an adjunctive treatment for modern minimally invasive procedures. The union of high-tech medicine and hypnosis, the oldest form of psychotherapy, would make for a happy marriage (D. Spiegel, 2006).

REFERENCES

Anbar, R. D. (2006). Enhancing the use of hypnosis in medical practice. *American Journal of Clinical Hypnosis, 49*(2), 97–99.

Anderson, K., & Masur, F. (1983). Psychological preparation for invasive medical and dental procedures. *Journal of Behavioral Medicine, 6*, 1–40.

Astin, J. A. (2004). Mind-body therapies for the management of pain. *Clinical Journal of Pain, 20*, 27–32.

Astin, J. A., Shapiro, S. L., Eisenberg, D. M., & Forys, K. L. (2003). Mind-body Medicine: State of the science, implications for practice. *Journal of the American Board of Family Practice, 16*, 131–147.

Baglini, R., Sesana, M., Capuano, C., Gnecchi-Ruscone, T., Ugo, L., & Danzi, G. B. (2004). Effect of hypnotic sedation during percutaneous transluminal coronary angioplasty on myocardial ischemia and cardiac sympathetic drive. *American Journal of Cardiology, 93*(8), 1035–1038.

Barabasz, A., & Christensen, C. (2006). Age regression: Tailored versus scripted inductions. *American Journal of Clinical Hypnosis, 48*(4), 251–261.

Barber, J. (1998). When hypnosis causes trouble. *International Journal of Clinical & Experimental Hypnosis, 46*, 157–170.

Blankfield, R. P. (1991). Suggestion, relaxation, and hypnosis as adjuncts in the care of surgery patients: A review of the literature. *American Journal of Clinical Hypnosis, 33*, 172–186.

Bugbee, M. E., Wellisch, D. K., Arnott, I. M., Maxwell, J. R., Kirsch, D. L., Sayre, J. W., et al. (2005). Breast core-needle biopsy: Clinical trial of relaxation technique versus medication versus no intervention for anxiety reduction. *Radiology, 234*, 73–78.

Butler, L. D., Symons, B. K., Henderson, S. L., Shortliffe, L. D., & Spiegel, D. (2005). Hypnosis reduces distress and duration of an invasive medical procedure for children. *Pediatrics, 115*, 77–85.

Campion, E. W. (1993). Why unconventional medicine? (editorial). *New England Journal of Medicine, 328*, 282–283.

Chung, F., Ritchie, E., & Su, J. (1997). Postoperative pain in ambulatory surgery. *Anesthesia Analgesia, 85*(4), 808–816.

Coe, W. C., & Ryken, K. (1979). Hypnosis and risks to human subjects. *American Psychologist, 34*(8), 673–681.

Duffy, J. (1964). Anglo-American reaction to obstetrical anesthesia. *Bulletin of the History of Medicine, 38*, 32–44.

Eisenberg, D. M., Kessler, R. C., Foster, C., Norlock, F. E., Calkins, D. R., & Delbanco, T. L. (1993). Unconventional medicine in the United States. *New England Journal of Medicine, 328*, 246–252.

Erickson III, J. C. (1994). The use of hypnosis in anesthesia: A master class commentary. *International Journal of Clinical & Experimental Hypnosis, 42*, 8–12.

Esdaile, J. (1846/1957). *Mesmerism in India and its practical application in surgery and medicine.* London. Re-issued as *Hypnosis in medicine and surgery.* New York (1957): Julian Press.

Faymonville, M. E., Fissette, J., Mambourg, P. H., Roediger, L., Joris, J., & Lamy, M. (1995). Hypnosis as adjunct therapy in conscious sedation for plastic surgery. *Regional Anesthesia, 20*, 145–151.

Faymonville, M. E., Laureys, S., Degueldre, C., et al. (2000). Neural mechanisms of antinociceptive effects of hypnosis. *Anesthesiology, 92*, 1257–67.

Fick, L. J., Lang, E. V., Benotsch, E. G., Lutgendorf, S., & Logan, H. L. (1999). Imagery content during nonpharmacologic analgesia in the procedure suite. Where your patients would rather be. *Academic Radiology, 6*, 457–463.

Flory, N., Salazar, G. M., & Lang, E. V. (2007). Hypnosis for acute distress management during medical procedures. *International Journal of Clinical & Experimental Hypnosis, 55*(3), 303–317.

Ghoneim, M. M., Block, R. I., Sarasin, D. S., Davis, C. S., & Marchman, J. N. (2000). Tape-recorded hypnosis instructions as adjuvant in the care of patients scheduled for third molar surgery. *Anesthesia Analgesia, 90*, 64–68.

Gracely, R. H., McGrath, P. A., Heft, M. W., & Dubner, R. (1977). Threshold and suprathreshold sensations produced by electrical tooth pulp stimuli and their modification by fentanyl, a narcotic analgesic. *Neuroscience Abstracts, 3*, 482.

Grant, G. J., Grant, A. H., & Lockwood, C. J. (2005). Simpson, Semmelweis, and transformational change. *Obstetrics & Gynecology, 106*(2), 384–387.

Hart, R. R. (1980). The influence of a taped hypnotic induction treatment procedure on the recovery of surgery patients. *International Journal of Clinical & Experimental Hypnosis, 28*(4), 324–332.

Hatsiopoulou, O., Cohen, R. I., & Lang, E. (2003). Postprocedure pain management of interventional radiology patients. *Journal of Vascular & Interventional Radiology, 14*, 1373–1385.

Huth, M. M., Broome, M. E., & Good, M. (2004). Imagery reduces children's postoperative pain. *Pain, 110*, 439–448.

Jensen, M. P., McArthur, K. D., Barber, J., Hanley, M. A., Engel, J. M., Romano, J. M., et al. (2006). Satisfaction with, and the beneficial side effects of, hypnotic analgesia. *International Journal of Clinical & Experimental Hypnosis, 54*(4), 432–447.

Jensen, M. P., & Patterson, D. R. (2005). Control conditions in hypnotic-analgesia clinical trials-Challenges and recommendations. *Journal of Clinical and Experimental Hypnosis, 53*, 170–197.

Jones, W. H. S. (1923/1972). *Hippocrates with an English translation.* Cambridge: Harvard University Press.

Lang, E. V., Benotsch, E. G., Fick, L. J., Lutgendorf, S., Berbaum, M. L., Berbaum, K. S., et al. (2000). Adjunctive non-pharmacologic analgesia for invasive medical procedures: a randomized trial. *Lancet, 355*, 1486–1490.

Lang, E. V., Berbaum, K. S., Faintuch, S., Hatsiopoulou, O., Halsey, N., Li, X., et al. (2006). Adjunctive self-hypnotic relaxation for outpatient medical procedures: A prospective randomized trial with women undergoing large core breast biopsy. *Pain, 126*, 155–164.

Lang, E. V., Chen, F., Fick, L. J., & Berbaum, K. S. (1998). Determinants of intravenous conscious sedation for arteriography. *Journal of Vascular & Interventional Radiology, 9*, 407–412.

Lang, E. V., Hatsiopoulou, O., Koch, T., Berbaum, K., Lutgendorf, S., Kettenmann, E., et al. (2005). Can words hurt? Patient-provider interactions during invasive procedures. *Pain, 114*(1–2), 303–309.

Lang, E. V., Joyce, J. S., Spiegel, D., Hamilton, D., & Lee, K. (1996). Self-hypnotic relaxation during interventional radiological procedures. Effects on pain perception and intravenous drug use. *International Journal of Clinical & Experimental Hypnosis, 44*, 106–119.

Lang, E. V., Lutgendorf, S., Logan, H., Benotsch, E., Laser, E., & Spiegel, D. (1999). Nonpharmacologic analgesia and anxiolysis for interventional radiological procedures. *Seminars in Interventional Radiology, 16*, 113–123.

Lang, E. V., & Rosen, M. (2002). Cost analysis of adjunct hypnosis for sedation during outpatient interventional procedures. *Radiology, 222*, 375–382.

Lutgendorf, S. K., Lang, E. V., Berbaum, K. S., Russell, D., Berbaum, M. L., Logan, H., et al. (2007). Effects of age on responsiveness to adjunct hypnotic analgesia during invasive medical procedures. *Psychosomatic Medicine, 69*(2), 191–199.

Lynn, S. J., Martin, D. J., & Frauman, D. C. (1996). Does hypnosis pose special risks for negative effects? A master class commentary. *International Journal of Clinical & Experimental Hypnosis, 44*, 7–19.

Mahnke, D., Chen, Y. K., Antillon, M. R., Brown, W. R., Mattison, R., & Shah, R. J. (2006). A prospective study of complications of endoscopic retrograde cholangiopancreatography and endoscopic ultrasound in an ambulatory endoscopy center. *Clinical Gastroenterology & Hepatology, 4*(7), 924–930.

Mander, R. (1998). A reappraisal of Simpson's introduction of chloroform. *Midwifery, 14*(3), 181–189.

Martin, M. L., & Lennox, P. H. (2003). Sedation and analgesia in the interventional radiology department. *Journal of Vascular & Interventional Radiology, 14*, 1119–1128.

Martin, M. L., Lennox, P. H., & Buckley, B. T. (2005). Pain and anxiety: Two problems, two solutions. *Journal of Vascular & Interventional Radiology, 16*, 1581–1584.

Melzack, R. (1999). Pain and stress: A new perspective. In R. J. Gatchel & D. C. Turk (Eds.), *Psychosocial factors in pain* (pp. 89–106). New York: Guilford Press.

Montgomery, G. H., Bovbjerg, D. H., Schnur, J. B., David, D., Goldfarb, A., Weltz, C. R., et al. (2007). A randomized clinical trial of a brief hypnosis intervention to control side effects in breast surgery patients. *Journal of the National Cancer Institute, 99*(17), 1304–1312.

Montgomery, G. H., David, D., Winkel, G., Silverstein, J. H., & Bovberg, D. H. (2002). The effectiveness of adjunctive hypnosis with surgical patients: A meta-analysis. *Anesthesia Analgesia, 94*, 1639–1645.

Morgan, A. H., & Hilgard, E. R. (1972). Age differences in susceptibility to hypnosis. *International Journal of Clinical & Experimental Hypnosis, 21*, 78–85.

Nuland, S. B. (2003). *The doctors' plague: Germs, childbed fever, and the strange story of Ignac Semmelweis* (pp. 98–99). New York: W.W. Norton.

Patterson, D. R., Questad, K. A., & deLateour, B. J. (1989). Hypnotherapy as an adjunct to narcotic analgesia for the treatment of pain for burn debridement. *American Journal of Clinical Hypnosis, 31*, 156–163.

Patterson, D. R., Hoffman, H. G., Palacios, A. G., Jensen, M. J. (2006) Analgesic effects of posthypnotic suggestions and virtual reality distraction on thermal pain. *Journal of Abnormal Psychology, 115*(4), 834–41.

Peteet, J. R., Stomper, P. C., Murray-Ross, D., Cotton, V., Truesdall, P., & Moczynski, W. (1992). Emotional support for patients with cancer who are undergoing CT: Semistructured interviews of patients at a cancer institute. *Radiology, 182*, 99–102.

Price, D. D., Harkins, S. W., & Baker, C. (1987). Sensory-affective relationships among different types of clinical and experimental pain. *Pain, 28*(3), 297–307.

Quirk, M. E., Letenre, A. J., Ciottone, R. A., & Lingley, J. F. (1989). Evaluation of three psychologic interventions to reduce anxiety during MR imaging. *Radiology, 173*, 759–762.

Rainville, P., Bao, Q. V. H., & Chretien, P. (2005). Pain-related emotions modulate experimental pain perception and autonomic responses. *Pain, 118*(3), 306–318.

Rainville, P., Carrier, B., Hofbauer, R. K., Bushnell, M. C., & Duncan, G. H. (1999). Dissociation of sensory and affective dimensions of pain using hypnotic modulation. *Pain, 82*, 159–171.

Rainville, P., Duncan, G. H., Price, D. D., Carrier, B., & Bushnell, M. C. (1997). Pain affect encoded in human anterior cingulate but not somatosensory cortex. *Science, 277*, 968–971.

Saadat, H. and Kain, Z. (2007). Hypnosis as a therapeutic tool. *Pediatrics*, *120*(1), 179–181.

Schupp, C., Berbaum, K., Berbaum, M., & Lang, E. V. (2005). Pain and anxiety during interventional radiological procedures. Effect of patients' state anxiety at baseline and modulation by nonpharmacologic analgesia adjuncts. *Journal of Vascular & Interventional Radiology*, *16*, 1585–1592.

Simpson, J. Y. (1847). Account of a new anaesthetic agent as a substitute for sulphuric ether in surgery and midwifery. Communications to the Medico-Chirurgical Society of Edinburgh 10th November. Edinburgh: Sutherland & Knox.

Skolnick, A. A. (1996). Sesquicentennial of first publicly performed surgery under anesthesia. *Journal of the American Medical Association*, *276*(15), 1205.

Spiegel, D. (2007). The mind prepared: hypnosis in surgery. *Journal of the National Cancer Institute*, *99*(17), 1280–1281.

Spiegel, D. (2006). Wedding hypnosis to the radiology suite. *Pain*, *126*(1–3), 3–4.

Spiegel, D., Bierre, P., & Rootenberg, J. (1989). Hypnotic alteration of somatosensory perception. *American Journal of Psychiatry*, *146*(6), 749–754.

Spiegel, D., & Bloom, J. (1983). Pain in metastatic breast cancer. *Cancer*, *52*, 341–345.

Spiegel, D., Detrick, D., & Frischolz, E. (1982). Hypnotizability and psychopathology. *American Journal of Psychiatry*, *139*, 431–437.

Spiegel, H. (1997). Nocebo: The power of suggestibility. *Preventive Medicine*, *26*, 616–621.

Spiegel, H., & Spiegel, D. (1978). *Trance and treatment: Clinical uses of hypnosis*. New York: Basic Books.

Stewart, J. H. (2005). Hypnosis in contemporary medicine. *Mayo Clinical Proceedings*, *80*, 511–524.

Wain, H. J. (2004). Reflections on hypnotizability and its impact on successful surgical hypnosis: A sole anesthetic for septoplasty. *American Journal of Clinical Hypnosis*, *46*(4), 313–321.

Wright, B. R., & Drummond, P. D. (2000). Rapid induction analgesia for the alleviation of procedural pain during burn care. *Burns*, *26*(3), 275–282.

Zeltzer, L., & LeBaron, S. (1982). Hypnosis and nonhypnotic techniques for reduction of pain and anxiety during painful procedures in children and adolescents with cancer. *Journal of Pediatrics*, *101*, 1032–1035.

This work was supported by the U.S. Army Medical Research and Material Command (DAMD 17-01-1-0153), National Institutes of Health & National Center for Complementary and Alternative Medicine (RO1 AT-0002-05 & K24 AT01074-01), Ruth L. Kirschstein National Research Service Award, National Institutes of Health & National Institute of Cancer (T32-59367).

Chapter 6

Hypnosis in the Treatment of Smoking, Alcohol, and Substance Abuse: The Nature of Scientific Evidence

Kent Cadegan and V. Krishna Kumar

The Substance and Mental Health Services Administration (2007) reported that in 2006, 72.9 million Americans (29.6 percent) aged 12 or older were current users (past month) of a tobacco product, the largest (61.6 million or 25 percent) were cigarette smokers. Furthermore, illicit drug use was almost 9 times higher (47.8 percent) among youths aged 12 to 17 who smoked cigarettes in the past month than it was among youths who did not smoke cigarettes in the past month (5.4 percent). Generally, illicit drug use was reported by 9.6 million persons aged 12 or older. Marijuana, a popular drug of choice of 14.8 million users, was smoked daily or almost daily over a period of 12 months by 3.1 million persons among past marijuana users, aged 12 or older. Heavy alcohol was reported by 17 million (6.9 percent) of the population aged 12 or older, or 17 million people, and binge drinking by 57 million people (23 percent). Even more troublesome is that in 2006, 10.2 million people (4.2 percent) aged 12 or older reported driving under the influence of illicit drugs during the past year.

Smoking is the leading contributor to premature death, cardiovascular disease, stroke, lung cancer, and, more recently, it has been linked to Alzheimer disease and dementia. A study of 6,868 people age 55 and older in the Netherlands, followed for seven years, showed current smokers, without an APOE ε4 allele, were at increased risk to develop Alzheimer dementia, than those who had never smoked. There was no association in whom the allele was present. There was, however, no association between current smoking and risk for vascular dementia, or past smoking and risk for dementia, Alzheimer dementia, and vascular dementia (Reitz, den Heijer, van Duijn, Hofman, & Breteler, 2007). Alcohol, cocaine opiates, other street and prescription drugs, and gambling wreak havoc in the lives of many people and stress the health care system, law enforcement, and employment agencies to a very high level in many developed countries. The social costs of addictions are indeed very high (Rehm, Taylor, Patra, & Gmel, 2006), given that there are multiple consequences of substance abuse—premature mortality, conflicts with family, unemployment, various psychiatric disorders, transmission of infectious diseases, automobile accidents, cancer, and a host of other medical ailments (Wagner et al., 2007).

Treatment options abound for people addicted to tobacco and illicit and prescription drugs. These include self-help groups such as Alcoholics Anonymous and Narcotics Anonymous; pharmacological interventions in the form of emetics, patches, and pills; acupuncture; and, psychological interventions that use behavioral, cognitive-behavioral, stress management, motivational, and hypnotic strategies to beat addictions. Of course, people often simultaneously attempt one or more interventions, for example acupuncture, patches, and cognitive-behavioral.

The rising cost of the dominant conventional allopathic system of pharmaceutical antidotes appears to be driving individuals to seek alternative systems of healing and wellness, including hypnosis. With over 300 alternative systems of health care the world over, it is necessary to establish the effectiveness of hypnosis as a treatment modality, particularly since it could be a very cost-effective treatment strategy. To think a simple daily self-hypnosis practice and timely hypnotherapy could offer significant relief begs more careful scrutiny than given Franz Mesmer by the French Academy of Sciences.

The purpose of this chapter is to review experimental evidence on the effectiveness of using hypnosis in the treatment of smoking and drug and alcohol abuse. The review is restricted to experimental work and is an examination of the Cochrane Database of Systematic Reviews (2000–2005), other past reviews, and recent individual experimental studies using hypnosis for the treatment of smoking, drug, and alcohol abuse.

HYPNOSIS IN THE TREATMENT OF SMOKING

Excellent reviews of literature (Holroyd, 1980; Green & Lynn, 2000; and most recently, Abbot, Stead, White, & Barnes, 2006) are already available on the impact of hypnosis on smoking cessation. They all paint a fairly grim picture about the effectiveness of hypnosis for smoking cessation with a minimal intervention of one or two sessions.

The reviews of Green and Lynn (2000) and Abbot et al. (2006) suggest that the most available studies suffer from one or more methodological weaknesses, thus failing to meet the criteria for meeting the highest levels of evidence for evidence-based research on the effectiveness of therapy. From a comprehensive review of clinical reports, nonrandomized/nonequivalent sample studies, experimental investigations with less than recommended sample size, and rigorous experimental studies, Green and Lynn

(2000) concluded: "giving hypnosis the stamp of a well-established treatment for smoking cessation is premature, although hypnosis can, with some justification, be regarded as a *possibly efficacious*, yet by no means specific, treatment for smoking cessation" (p. 216).

In a review on the effectiveness of a variety of smoking cessation interventions, Marlow and Stoller (2003) highlighted Abbot, Stead, White, Barnes, and Ernst (2000), finding no "efficacy of hypnosis for smoking cessation" (p. 1251), noting that the main challenges to validating the efficacy of hypnosis had to do with "small sample size of most of the trials and confounding issue of separating the impact of time spent with the therapist from the hypnosis itself" (p. 1251). Furthermore, they observed that "The USDHHS Clinical Practice Guideline do not recommend hypnosis" (p. 1251).

There is little evidence that hypnosis for smoking cessation does any better than other treatments (relaxation, behavior modification, and health education), attention, or placebo comparisons (see also Covino & Bottari, 2001). Re-examining the data reported by Green and Lynn (2000; Table 1), the median abstinence rates in clinical reports using 3, 6, and 12 months time frames were found to be 29, 25, and 19 percent, respectively. Furthermore, data on nonrandomized/nonequivalent sample studies, abstinence rates reported in Table 2 by Green & Lynn (2000) ranged from 1 month to 19 months in 5 very different studies, making it difficult to evaluate the effect of hypnosis in terms of specific time frames on abstinence rates. The median abstinence rate for hypnosis alone, for these varied time frames, was about 22 percent. The median abstinence rate was 31.5 percent for experimental studies with less than recommended sample size, using individual and group hypnosis conditions and using follow-up periods of 1 week to 6 months (based on Table 3, Green & Lynn, 2000). The median abstinence rate was 21 percent for follow-up time periods of 3 weeks to 6 months in rigorous experimental studies (estimates based on Table 3, Green & Lynn, 2000).

Abbot et al. (2006) considered only those studies that used randomized controlled trials that reported abstinence over at least 6 months after the beginning of the treatment. They found only nine such studies (through search of various data bases, 1966–2005) from which they concluded: (a) there was wide variation of results in individual studies, with conflicting results about the effectiveness of hypnosis, relative to other treatments or control conditions (wait listed/no treatment control, attention/placebo, psychological treatments, rapid/focused smoking, hypnosis plus group therapy vs. group therapy alone), (b) there was no evidence of a greater effect of hypnotherapy on 6-month abstinence rates, compared to other treatments or no treatment, (c) studies used a wide range of hypnotherapies, but did not describe them fully, (d) none of the studies used biochemical markers for determining abstinence at follow-up, (e) the increased likelihood of abstinence, in studies reporting success, may be due to non-specific factors such as contact with a therapist, and (f) the encouraging results from uncontrolled studies may be due to the inclusion of highly motivated participants and may not be reflective of long-term abstinence.

A recent study by Elkins and Rajab (2004) used a non-randomized control group study. The control was a consult-only group of nine patients (who chose not to participate after session 1) who were compared with patients who had experienced one ($n = 9$) or two sessions ($n = 12$) of hypnosis treatment. During the second session, patients were provided with a cassette tape (direct suggestions for relaxation and comfort) following hypnosis with individually adapted hypnosis suggestions at the end of the second session and were asked to practice four or more times per week. Although encouraging results were reported (48 percent abstinence rate at one year post-treatment), no results pertaining to the use of practice or its effects were reported.

Elkins, Marcus, Bates, Rajab, and Cook (2006) noted that many of the randomized studies have used "a minimal approach to hypnotherapy, involving one or two sessions or group interventions" yielding "outcomes about 20% to 25% cessation" (p. 304). Elkins et al. (2006) conducted a prospective randomized control group pilot study, involving intensive hypnotherapy for smoking cessation involving eight sessions, in which hypnotic interventions were conducted in sessions 1, 2, 4, and 7. Individualized suggestions were embedded in general common suggestions (across all subjects) of "deepening relaxation, absorbing in relaxing imagery, commitment to stop smoking, decreased craving for nicotine, posthypnotic suggestions, practice of self-hypnosis, and visualization of the positive benefits of smoking cessation" (p. 307). The 20 participants in the experimental group were also provided with self-help materials from the National Cancer Institute and brief counseling each session, plus a self-hypnosis tape recording and tape player and instructed in the daily practice of self-hypnosis. The participants also received supportive phone calls three days after the target quit date, and in weeks 2, 4, and 5. The 20 participants in the wait-listed group received self-help material, were encouraged to set a quit date, and received supportive phone calls. Using biochemical markers, they reported a 40 percent continuous abstinence rate (from quitting date) for the hypnosis participants as opposed to zero percent in the control group. Unfortunately, again, the study did not examine either the effects of hypnotic susceptibility or the effects of practice.

Lynn and Kirsch (2006) described a two-session program approach, using cognitive-behavioral training in conjunction with self-hypnosis training. Their program included the following components: self-hypnosis training, cognitive-behavioral skills, education, enhancing motivation and self-efficacy, being a nonsmoker, relapse prevention and gain maintenance, minimizing weight gain, and contracting and social support. They reported continuous abstinence rates of 24 to 39 percent at six-month follow-up ($n = 236$) across different trainers.

HYPNOSIS IN THE TREATMENT OF ALCOHOL AND SUBSTANCE ABUSE

Relative to smoking, very few experimental studies exist on the use of hypnosis in the treatment of alcohol and even fewer on substance abuse, although there appears to be a growing interest in using hypnosis for treating alcoholism and other addictions (Potter, 2004). Early reviews by Wadden and Penrod (1981), Wadden and Anderton (1982), and Schoen (1985) suggest mixed findings. Experimental studies showed little effects of hypnosis on alcohol abstinence, but case studies reported encouraging results. All reviews pointed to various methodological flaws in the reviewed studies that make it highly problematic to conclude that hypnosis qualifies as an evidence-based approach (or even possibly efficacious) for treating alcohol abuse. Examining more current literatures suggests that this has not changed. There have been a few dissertations on the adjunctive usefulness of hypnosis (Chierici, 1989; Crocker, 2004; Smith, 1988; Young, 1996) in the treatment of alcohol abuse. Unfortunately, none of these studies say much about the efficacy of hypnosis as an evidence-based approach, either as an adjunctive technique or as stand-alone treatment strategy in the treatment of alcohol abuse or dependence. They worked with small sample sizes, short-follow-up time frames (1 week to 90 days), and outcomes were assessed via self-report.

As mentioned before, experimental studies with substance abuse patients are even more rare. A recent randomized controlled trial by Pekala et al. (2004) was a step in this direction. They used random assignment across four conditions (hypnosis, transtheoretical, cognitive-behavioral, and attention-placebo labeled as stress management conditions). All 261 veterans included in the study were involved in either a 21 or 28 (dual diagnosis) substance abuse day treatment program involving intensive group and individual therapy five days a week, approximately six hours a day. The veterans received an additional four hours of training in self-hypnosis, a cognitive-behavioral transtheoretical intervention (based on Prochaska, Norcross, & DiClemente, 1992), or an attention-placebo (stress management) intervention program. Thus, the treatment conditions in the study were all adjunctive to the regular domiciliary programs. The veterans received treatment manuals in the four conditions, which they could refer to use and use on a regular basis during treatment and postdischarge.

The hypnosis treatment included four hypnosis protocols: self-esteem enhancement, relapse prevention, serenity enhancement, and anger and anxiety reduction/management. The relapse prevention hypnotic protocol used suggestions based on H. Spiegel (1970) and suggestions for relapse prevention based on Marlatt and Gordon (1985). All protocols included body-scan relaxation and mind-calming suggestions. The participants were encouraged to practice "whatever self-hypnosis protocol they wanted, but to do so at least once per day for the next 3 months" (p. 285). A two-month self-report follow-up was conducted. Of the 54 percent of participants contacted, 87 percent reported total abstinence in all four groups. While there were no significant overall differences in the four experimental conditions in relapse rates, possibly due to the excellent residential program everyone received, some interesting findings did emerge, "with severely addicted individuals, practicing self-hypnosis tapes regularly (at least 4 times a week) postdischarge was associated with increased self-esteem and serenity, and decreased anger impulsivity" (p. 292). Additionally, "participants were more likely to be abstinent to the extent they practiced the audiotapes, and at the beginning of the study had lower levels of self-esteem, were already practicing counter-conditioning strategies, and did not practice stimulus control" (p. 293).

Given that hypnotic responsivity was associated with those who practiced the self-hypnosis tapes, the results suggest a specific mediating effect of hypnosis. The study's results can be considered encouraging as an evidence-based adjunctive treatment strategy, in as much as it suggests the use of multiple hypnotic protocols and the significance of self-hypnosis practice for more hypnotically responsive patients. Although the study used random assignment, treatment manuals, and had adequate sample size in each condition, the follow-up relied upon self-reports, and the number of individuals available for final analyses were small. Unfortunately, the data on what protocols were actually practiced were not collected, thus it is not possible to determine what mechanisms were actually at work in the participants who found hypnosis helpful.

GENERAL DISCUSSION

Examining both extant reviews and recent experimental studies on the use of hypnosis for smoking cessation suggests that the conclusion of Green and Lynn (2000) of hypnosis as a *"possibly efficacious,* yet by no means specific, treatment for smoking cessation" (p. 216) still remains valid. If a potential client calls and asks, does it work, we are still unable to give a clear substantive answer as to what would be a reasonable expectation of success. Given abstinence rates of zero to 88 percent in different studies, even with rather gross estimates of about 20 percent success rates, it is not clear what statement can be made to a potential client as to what to expect. In contrast, it is noteworthy that Law and Tang (1995) reported that an estimated 2 percent of smokers stopped smoking and did not relapse up to a year as a result of brief unsolicited advice from their physician, leading them to conclude that although the effect is modest, this is a very cost-effective strategy. It would be interesting to determine if physician-referred patients for hypnosis are more successful than those referred from other sources (e.g., friends, families, self).

The conclusion with regard to the use of treatment of alcohol and drugs is even bleaker, despite the number of good ideas that are available in the designing of hypnotic treatment protocols and tested in somewhat less rigorous studies that suggest that hypnotic strategies are valuable for at least some clients.

Some key recommendations emerge from a review of these various studies. There is a need to standardize the measurement of outcomes by way of using biochemical markers. There appears to be an over-reliance on the more conveniently obtained self-report measures. Follow-up intervals tend to be short, possibly because of inadequate funding of such projects and perhaps also the increasing difficulty of maintaining contacts over time with the participants. However, there is a need for systematizing the follow-up intervals in different studies. Possibly the minimal requirement for such outcome studies should use follow-up time frames of 3, 6, and 12 months. With increasingly long-term follow-ups, there is an increasing problem for internal validity, in as much as there is a potential for greater within-conditions variability (Westen, Novotny, & Thomson-Brenner, 2004). Investigators should also report whether the participants were continuously abstinent over the time frames used in the study, along with frequency of lapses and relapses, and not just whether they were abstinent at the single point of time at follow-up. A study of lapses and how participants recover from lapses would be valuable. There is also a need to evaluate the effectiveness of hypnosis for different types of smokers—light, medium, or heavy—and chronic (hardened smokers) versus those have smoked for a short period of time.

In designing studies, one needs to employ a hypnosis-alone condition, along with hypnosis-plus another treatment such as cognitive-behavioral, cognitive-behavioral alone, and an attention-placebo condition to more accurately assess the role of hypnosis as an adjunctive technique. The question of how many sessions do we need remains to be addressed. There is a need to systematically examine the popular one-session approach with a more multiple-session approach, especially in view of the popular one-large group sessions that are offered by lay hypnotists in hotels around the country. Studies are needed to examine the effectiveness of particular suggestions used in hypnosis protocols. This can be done by both asking patients what they found most helpful in the hypnotic protocol used and more rigorously by conducting controlled experiments. Yet another possibility is to examine if stages of change (Prochaska et al., 1992) are important in the type of suggestions used. Such analyses will be helpful in making specific recommendations to clinicians. Currently, a wide range of suggestions are used and it is not known what suggestions are particularly helpful and when (i.e., in terms of stages of change). In studies where multiple protocols are used, addressing tangential, but relevant aspects, such as improving self-esteem, reducing anger (e.g., Pekala et al., 2004), it is important to follow up on understanding their contribution to the treatment process.

Studies are needed to examine the effectiveness of individualizing suggestions versus using pre-scripted versions and their association with hypnotizability. The chief advantage of pre-scripted protocols is that they can be administered by a minimally trained technician and/or via audiotapes. In contrast, individualized protocols clearly require experience and would require individual taping. Hypnotizability needs to be routinely assessed in treatment outcome studies, as Bowers (1984) noted "the effects of a treatment intervention are not due to a suggestion *unless* treatment outcome is correlated with hypnotic ability" (p. 444), the point of view is referred to as the "Bowers Doctrine" (Woody, 1997, p. 227).

Pekala et al.'s study suggests the importance of self-hypnosis practice (see also Potter, 2004). However, not much is known about the role of self-hypnosis practice as it relates to treatment outcomes. Specifically, how much practice is needed and for how long? Is distributed practice better than massed practice? Is it better to use taped scripts or have the patients practice without audiotapes on self-generated suggestions? And, is there a role for hypnosis booster sessions in maintenance?

Since hypnosis is popularly sought as treatment of smoking cessation, it is imperative that studies are urgently needed to not just establish it as an effective treatment, but also to determine the essential components of a hypnotic intervention. Thus, there is a need to know what works and what does not work and for whom (i.e., types of suggestions, types of practice, individual vs. group, types of adjunctive treatment, individually tailored vs. pre-scripted versions, influence of individual difference variables; see Spiegel, Frischholz, Fleiss, & Spiegel, 1993).

There is indeed a significant body of work (case studies, quasi-experimental studies, and experimental studies) that suggests hypnosis is a viable treatment option, and there is no dearth of good ideas about how hypnotic protocols are to be designed—but there is a need for testing these ideas using experimental methods. Eventually, it should be possible to say to a potential client that hypnosis can help you control your addiction if you have certain characteristics (e.g., hypnotizability, motivation to quit; availability of social support), and if you are willing to practice (with specification about the nature and amount of practice).

There is no exclusive methodology by which science progresses—there is a place for a variety of different types of methodologies, informing one another. On a cautionary note, it is important to realize that the randomized controlled trials, the "gold standard" (Cooper, 2003, p. 106) of evidence-based practice, has weaknesses. Most importantly, such trials address narrow issues, use carefully selected samples, use short-trial periods, and provide information about a group, not individual treatment (see Cooper, 2003; Williams & Garner, 2002), among other problems. Williams and Garner (2002) pointed out that even a single successfully treated patient might provide information on a breakthrough procedure, for example, "the first surgical operation for mitral stenosis" (p. 11). Thus, evidence that is based on randomized controlled trials is not to be construed as a guarantee of success in practice At best, they provide guidance and needs to combine with clinical experience for making treatment decisions. Williams and Garner (2002) noted: "Sophisticated clinical experience with regard to an individual patient needs to be balanced with an evidence base derived from a group. Too much emphasis on a narrow range of acceptable evidence oversimplifies the complex nature of clinical care" (p. 11). Furthermore, even well-established medical practices do not always work for everyone. And, what may generally not work may have extraordinary effects in some individuals. Williams and Garner (2002) observed: "The EBM [Evidence-Based Medicine] data on donezpil show marginal improvement in patients with mild to moderate dementia. On the other hand, there are good examples of individual patients showing impressive improvement in patients (Dening & Lawton, 1998; Manchip & Morrison, 1999). Evidence of this nature must be recognized and not dismissed as anecdotal (p. 10)."

A recent exciting finding was reported by Naqvi, Rudrauf, Damasio, & Bechara (2007) concerning the role of the insula in controlling conscious urges for nicotine. Damage to the insula was accompanied by "disruption of smoking addiction, characterized by the ability to quit smoking easily, immediately, without relapse, and without persistence of the urge to smoke" (p. 531). A patient who had smoked "40 unfiltered cigarettes per day and was enjoying smoking very much" (p. 534) quit smoking immediately after suffering a stroke; he stated "he quit because his 'body' forgot the urge to smoke" (p. 534), suggesting that smoking serves to satisfy a bodily need. In a media report, one of the authors of the study, Bechara, stated: "The quitting was like a light switch turned off and he never wanted a cigarette again" (Dunham, 2007, pp. 1–2). Naqvi et al. (2007) suggested that "therapies that modulate the function of insula will be useful in helping smokers quit" (p. 534) Well, can hypnosis practitioners design suggestions to turn odown the insula when faced with cravings, or, to gain greater control by being able to turn it up and down volitionally?

REFERENCES

Abbot, N. C., Stead, L. F., White, A. R., & Barnes, J. (2006). Hypnotherapy for Smoking Cessation. *The Cochrane Database for Systematic Reviews*, the Cochrane Library, the Cochrane Collaboration, Volume 4. Retrieved November 17, 2006, from http://grateway.ut.ovoid.com/gw1/0vidweb.cgi.

Abbot, N. C., Stead, L. F., White, A. R., Barnes, J., & Ernst, E. (2000). Hypnotherapy for Smoking Cessation. *The Cochrane Database for Systematic Reviews*, the Cochrane Library, the Cochrane Collaboration, Volume 2.

Bowers, K. S. (1984). Hypnosis. In N. S. Endler & J. M. Hunt (Eds.), *Personality and the behavioral disorders* (pp. 23–54). Washington, DC: American Psychological Association.

Chierici, S. (1989). The use of hypnosis to increase self-concept with drug and alcohol abusers. Dissertation Abstracts International, 50, 1676 (University Microfilm No. 8912409).

Cooper, B. (2003). Evidence-based mental health policy: A critical appraisal. *British Journal of Psychiatry, 183*, 105–113.

Covino, N. A., & Bottari, M. (2001). Hypnosis, behavioral theory, and smoking cessation. *Journal of Dental Education, 65*, 340–347.

Crocker, S. M. (2004). *Hypnosis as an adjunct in the treatment of alcohol relapse.* Unpublished dissertation, Washington State University, Washington.

Dening, T., & Lawton, C. (1998). New drug treatment to Alzheimer's disease. *British Medical Journal, 317*, 945.

Dunham, W. (2007). Brain damage makes heavy smoker quit. *News in Science abc. net.au/science/news.* Retrieved January 26, 2007 from http://www.abc.net.au. science/2007/1834202.htm/.

Green, J. P., & Lynn, S. J. (2000). Hypnosis and suggestion-based approaches to smoking cessation: An examination of the evidence. *International Journal of Clinical and Experimental Hypnosis, 48*, 195–224.

Elkins, G., Marcus, J., Bates, J., Rajab, M. H., & Cook, T. (2006). Intensive hypnotherapy for smoking cessation. *International Journal of Clinical and Experimental Hypnosis, 54*, 303–315.

Elkins, G., & Rajab, M. H. (2004). Clinical hypnosis for smoking cessation: Preliminary results of a three-session intervention. *International Journal of Clinical and Experimental Hypnosis, 52*, 73–84.

Green, J. P., Lynn, S. J. (2000). Hypnosis and suggestion-based approaches to smoking cessation. *International Journal of Clinical and Experimental Hypnosis, 48*(2), 195–223.

Holroyd, J. (1980). Hypnosis treatment for smoking: An evaluative review. *International Journal of Clinical and Experimental Hypnosis, 28*, 341–357.

Law, M., & Tang, J. L. (1995). An analysis of the effectiveness of interventions intended to help people stop smoking. *Archives of Internal Medicine, 155*, 1933–1941.

Lynn, S. J. & Kirsch, I. (2006). *Essentials of clinical hypnosis: An evidence based approach.* Washington, D.C.: American Psychological Association.

Manchip, S., & Morrison, C. (1999). A case report. *British Medical Journal, 139*, 1510.

Marlatt, G. A., & Gordon, J. R., (1985). *Relapse prevention: Maintenance strategies in the treatment of addictive behaviors.* New York: Guilford.

Marlow, S. P., & Stoller, J. K. (2003). Smoking cessation. *Respiratory Care, 48*, 1238–1256.

Naqvi, N. H., Rudrauf, D., Damasio, H., & Bechara, A. (2007). Damage to the insula disrupts addiction to cigarette smoking. *Science, 315*, 531–534.

Pekala, R. J., Maurer, R., Kumar, V.K., Elliott, N.C., Masten, E., & Moon, E. et al. (2004). Self-hypnosis relapse prevention training: Its effects on self-esteem, affect, and relapse with drug and alcohol users. *American Journal of Clinical Hypnosis, 46*, 281–297.

Potter, G. (2004). Intensive therapy: Utilizing hypnosis in the treatment of substance abuse disorders. *American Journal of Clinical Hypnosis, 47*, 21–28.

Prochaska, J. O., Norcross, J. C., & DiClemente, C. (1992). In search of how people change. *American Psychologist, 47*, 1102–1114.

Rehm, J., Taylor, B., Patra, J., & Gmel, G. (2006). Avoidable burden of disease: Conceptual and methodological issues in substance abuse epidemiology. *International Journal of Methods in Psychiatric Research, 15,* 181–191.

Reitz, C., den Heijer, T., Van Duijn, C., Hofman, A., & Breteler, M. M. B. (2007). Relation between smoking and risk of dementia and Alzheimer disease. *Neurology, 69,* 998–1005.

Schoen, M. (1985). A conceptual framework and treatment strategy for the alcoholic urge to drink utilizing hypnosis. *International Journal of Addictions, 20,* 403–415.

Smith, M. B. (1988). The hypnotic modification of alcohol expectancies. *Dissertation Abstracts International, 49,* 5034 (University Microfilm No. 8903527).

Spiegel, D., Frischholz, E. J., Fleiss, J. L., & Spiegel, H. (1993). Predictors of smoking abstinence following a single-session restructuring intervention with self-hypnosis. *American Journal of Psychiatry, 150,* 1090–1097.

Spiegel, H. (1970). A single treatment method to stop smoking using ancillary self-hypnosis. *International Journal of Clinical and Experimental Hypnosis, 18,* 235–250.

Substance and Mental Health Services Administration (2007). *Results from the 2006 National Survey on Drug Use and health: National Findings.* Office of Applied Statistics, NSDUH Series H-32, DHHS Publication No. SMA 07-4293, Rockville, MD.

Wadden, T. A., & Anderton, C. H. (1982). The clinical use of hypnosis. *Psychological Bulletin, 91,* 215–243.

Wadden, T. A., & Penrod, J. H. (1981). Hypnosis in the treatment of alcoholism: A review and appraisal. *American Journal of Clinical Hypnosis, 24,* 41–47.

Wagner, T. H., Harris, K. M., Federman, B., Dei, L., & Luna, Y., & Humphreys, K. (2007). Prevalence of substance use disorders among veterans and comparable nonveterans from the national survey on drug use and health. *Psychological Services, 4,* 149–157.

Westen, D., Novotny, C. M., & Thomson-Brenner, H. (2004). The empirical status of empirically supported psychotherapies: Assumptions, findings, and reporting in controlled clinical trials. *Psychological Bulletin, 130,* 631–633.

Williams, D. D. R., & Garner, J. (2002). The case against "the evidence": A different perspective on evidence-based medicine. *British Journal of Psychiatry, 180,* 8–12.

Woody, E. Z. (1997). Have the hypnotically susceptibility scales outlived their usefulness? *International Journal of Clinical and Experimental Hypnosis, 45,* 226–238.

Young, G. K. (1996). *Hypnosis as an adjunctive modality in the relapse prevention component of an alcoholism treatment program.* Unpublished doctoral dissertation, Pacific Graduate School of Psychology, Palo Alto.

AUTHORS' NOTE

The authors thank Dr. R. J. Pekala for his comments on an earlier version of this chapter. Reprint requests are to be addressed to V. K. Kumar, Department of Psychology, West Chester University of Pennsylvania, West Chester, PA 19393; e-mail: vkumar@wcupa.edu

Chapter 7

Hypnosis and Medicine: In from the Margins

Nicholas A. Covino, Jessica Wexler, and Kevin Miller

A significant relationship between psychological variables, most notably anxiety and depression, has been found to be present in a variety of medical illnesses (Roy-Byrne et al. 2008). Psychological interventions in medicine commonly employ cognitive-behavioral and relaxation strategies that target the autonomic nervous system and improve social support for patients. Behavioral medicine strategies seek to manage increases in heart rate, respiration, muscle tension, and the overproduction of glucose, neurotransmitters, and hormones that result from sustained sympathetic arousal and benefit patients with pain, insomnia, asthma, gastrointestinal disorders, and some others (Giardion, McGrady, & Andrasik, 2007). Cognitive processes are thought to play a key role in the maintenance of these medical illnesses and somewhat in their treatment (Grossman, Neimann, Schmit, & Walach, 2004; Lehrer, Carr, Sargunaraj, & Woolfolk, 1993). Social supports are purported to provide emotional and instrumental assistance for patients and contribute beneficially to longevity (Anderson, 2003).

Hypnosis interventions with pain patients have been found, in varying degrees, to be efficacious (Montgomery, DuHamel, & Redd, 2000; Patterson & Jensen, 2003). Reviews of the hypnosis literature and in other areas propose that medical illness and conditions such as insomnia, asthma, bulimia, and irritable bowel syndrome and illness behaviors such as cigarette smoking and hyperemesis point to opportunities for symptom reduction and illness management via hypnosis (Covino, 2008; Mendoza & Capafons, 2009; Pinnel & Covino, 2000). Recent research with children and adults who are undergoing painful medical procedures supports the use of hypnosis as a distraction and pain management technique not only to decrease discomfort, but also, the use of medication and the time required for treatment (Butler, Symons, Henderson, Shortliffe & Spiegel, 2005; Lang et al., 2000).

Hypnotic interventions have a long history in the treatment of the medically ill. However, apart from the role of hypnosis in pain management, much of the research support for the use of hypnosis with the medically ill is dated or lacks sufficient methodological rigor to qualify for recommendation as an adjunct to medical care by mainstream practitioners. Most limiting are the parochial experimental models and idiosyncratic treatment protocols of hypnosis that ignore the research findings of other psychology and behavioral medicine investigators. The hypnosis literature on pain management provides significant reason to believe that hypnotic techniques can be of benefit to medical patients (Patterson & Jensen, 2003) and that there is some support for its extension to other illness areas (Pinnel & Covino, 2000). However, methodological weaknesses in the hypnosis literature, such as absent or dated research, a paucity of randomized control experiments, and the common failure of hypnosis researchers to integrate the results of studies from behavioral science investigators and other medical research, limit the acceptance of hypnosis as an adjunctive technique by patients and professionals. Advancement in this area seems achievable, but greater recognition requires the hypnosis community to update its literature, integrate findings from other researchers in psychology and medicine, and bring increased methodological rigor to research strategies to accomplish this.

Several medical illnesses and conditions serve as good examples of the promise and challenge for hypnosis in medicine, and these will be reviewed in this chapter. Since the efficacious role of hypnosis in pain management is best established and has been the subject of several excellent analyses (Montgomery, DuHamel, & Redd, 2000; Patterson & Jensen, 2003) we will not discuss it in further detail in this chapter.

ABSENT RESEARCH SUPPORT: INSOMNIA

Between 40 and 70 million Americans experience at least one episode of sleeplessness each year with chronic insomnia claiming about 20 percent of the adult population and close to 30 percent of those in senior years (Foley et al., 1995; NIH, 2005). Psychophysiologic insomnia is second in frequency only to the complaint of pain among primary care patients (Hauri & Linde, 1996) and it is the result of the combination of autonomic nervous system (ANS) arousal and injudicious behavior.

Consistent with a pattern of chronic ANS arousal, insomniacs use increased oxygen during the day and at night (Bonnet & Arand, 2003); demonstrate persistent elevations in temperature, heart rate, basal skin response, and vasoconstriction prior to and during sleep (Bonnet & Arand, 1998; Lushington, Dawson, & Lack, 2000); and report more frequent pre-sleep negative cognitive activity (Harvey, 2000; Kuisk, Bertelson, & Walsh, 1989; Nelson & Harvey,

2003). In an effort to cope with chronic insomnia, individuals commonly self-medicate with alcohol, establish irregular sleep habits, and engage in behaviors such as reading and watching television in bed that are incompatible with sleep. A repetitive cycle of arousal that includes catastrophic thinking, increased cardiopulmonary activity, maladaptive behaviors, and the release of hormones and neurotransmitters maintains the disorder. Sedative medications are sometimes prescribed, but psychological treatments such as cognitive behavioral therapy (CBT) that emphasize relaxation, cognitive restructuring (e.g., challenging and revising catastrophic thinking, such as "I must get to sleep soon or I will have a terrible day tomorrow.") and "sleep hygiene" (e.g., regularizing bedtime, avoiding daytime naps, leaving the bed when sleep is delayed more than 20 minutes), are recommended treatments (NIH, 2005).

Seventy-eight adults with chronic insomnia who were randomly assigned to receive medication (Temazepam), CBT, CBT + medication, or placebo reported better results for all active treatment conditions. While the best results were obtained by patients in the combined condition, CBT not only outperformed the medication-alone group, but, at one- and two-year follow-up, subjects reported greater relief and satisfaction with the psychological intervention over medication alone (Morin, Colecchi, Stone, Sood, & Brink, 1999). In a double-blind, placebo, controlled study, patients who were offered six weeks of CBT increased their hours of sleep and reduced the time that it took to fall asleep more than those trained with relaxation alone or subjected to desensitization techniques (Edinger et al., 2001). When insomnia patients were, again, randomly assigned to treatment conditions that included CBT, placebo, a popular sleep medication, and the combination medicine and CBT, both of the cognitive interventions had significant effect at six months on sleep efficiency over placebo and medication alone (Jacobs, Pace-Schott, Stickgold, & Otto, 2004). Patients who were offered the psychological intervention reported greater satisfaction with their results than those in the medication group. Interestingly, this type of cognitive-behavioral intervention has been found to be equally successful whether it is administered in a group, individually, or over the telephone in a 20-minute format (Bastien, Morin, Ouellet, Blais, & Bouchard, 2004).

A National Institute of Health expert panel, charged with reviewing the state of the science on insomnia, concluded that cognitive and behavioral techniques were the most effective psychological interventions for this disorder (NIH, 2005). Unfortunately, hypnosis was *not* recommended by the committee, due to a lack of available evidence in support of it. Although this aptly named (i.e., ύπνοσ = sleep, from the Greek) technique captures attention, facilitates absorption, alters perception, and offers suggestions for cognitive and behavioral change, researchers have not subjected it to empirical trials. It is easy to hypothesize that those who are blessed with vivid imaginations could be more susceptible to sleep disruption. Furthermore, this same capacity for absorption and imaginative involvement seems likely to permit patients with hypnosis to relax deeply and distract themselves from arousing thoughts in a manner that would facilitate sleep. However, *only anecdotal case reports exist* for hypnotic interventions with sleep-disordered patients, making it impossible to include among the evidence-based treatments in medicine.

DATED RESEARCH SUPPORT: ASTHMA, BULIMIA, HYPEREMESIS

Asthma

Asthma is a chronic medical illness that is characterized by episodes of inflammation and narrowing of the small airways of the lung, leading to symptoms of wheezing, shortness of breath, cough, and chest tightness. Approximately 22 million people in the United States suffer from asthma, and this number has been rising significantly due to lifestyle issues such as obesity, pollution, and smoking (Yeatts et al., 2006; National Heart Lung and Blood Institute 2008). Asthma results in lost work days and health care costs that exceed $16 billion per year and is among the most common causes of absenteeism among school-age children (NHLBI, 2008). Asthmatic episodes are commonly triggered by allergens, infection, and exercise, but psychological factors such as anxiety and panic are thought to be triggers as well (Kayton, Richardson, Lozano, & McCauley, 2004).

For many years, bronchial asthma was regarded as a "psychosomatic" illness. Early psychoanalysts (Alexander & French 1945; French & Alexander, 1941) grouped asthma among seven illnesses, including ulcerative colitis and neurodermatitis, where psychological conflicts were determined to be necessary and sufficient causes of disease. The asthma patient's signature wheeze was seen as a symbolic expression of dependency (i.e., "a suppressed cry for help from the mother") that would be resolved, along with the medical illness, by psychoanalysis. Later work in the 1970s, influenced by an understanding of asthma as a "hyperreactive airways disease" where the smooth muscle surrounding airways in the lung becomes triggered by heightened emotion, identified anxiety as an emotional trigger for an asthma attack. Susceptible individuals would not only be more vulnerable to increased symptoms but characterological anxiety was found to negatively impact the management and course of care (Jones, Kinsman, Dirks, & Dahlem, 1979; Kinsman, Dirks, Jones, & Dahlem, 1980). More recent studies continue to find a relationship between panic disorder and asthma sufferers. Hasler and her colleagues found that children with panic disorder were six times more likely to develop asthma as adults, and that asthmatic children were found to have a 4.5-fold incidence of panic disorder as adults (Hasler et al., 2005). The World Mental Health Survey of more than 85,000 adults found that asthma patients were 1.5 times more likely than non-asthmatics to experience panic and related anxiety disorders (Scott et al.,

2007). The more recent medical understanding of asthma as an inflammatory disease that is regulated by the immune system has invited researchers in the emerging field of "psychoneuroimmunology" to examine the relationship among psychological stress, immune response, and asthma symptomatology (Wright, 2004).

Early research utilizing suggestion and hypnosis in the treatment of asthma produced a rationale to include it in asthma care and some measure of hope for its efficacy. An experimental model, developed in the mid-1960s, measured airways resistance among asthmatics exposed to saline mist who were given "suggestions" that they were breathing bronchoconstricting irritants. Nineteen of 40 asthmatics reacted to the experimental situation with a significant increase in airways resistance and 12 of the asthmatic subjects developed full-blown attacks of bronchospasm that was reversed with a saline solution placebo (Luparello, Lyons, Bleecker, & McFadden, 1968). A meta-analysis of 23 studies that followed this same model found that one-third of the total 427 subjects in these studies demonstrated clinically significant responses to suggestions for breathing difficulties.

Two randomized, control studies are some of the best work in this area and each is more than 40 years old (British Tuberculosis Association, 1968; Maher-Loughnan, Mason, Macdonald, & Fry, 1962). At 18 months, asthma patients with hypnosis training demonstrated a significant decrease in medication use over asthma patient-controls without such training (Maher-Loughnan et al., 1962). A large sample ($N = 252$) randomized clinical trial examined the efficacy of relaxation training alone versus monthly hypnosis training with daily practice and found improvements in both groups. However, significantly better reduction in symptoms and medication use, especially among female patients, was noted for those in the hypnosis condition (British Tuberculosis Association, 1968). Patients with heightened hypnotizability were found to benefit from a supportive visit, but experienced significantly more benefit when trained to use hypnosis to manage asthma symptoms (Ewer & Stewart, 1986). A small group of 10 patients with exercise-induced asthma performed significantly better on treadmill tests when trained to use hypnosis than when they were offered a medication, a placebo, or standard care (Ben-Zvi, Spohn, Young, & Kattan, 1982). A more recent study (Anbar, 2002) found improvement for 80 percent of children who were offered hypnosis training, but it is unclear whether these children were asthmatic or were "pseudo-asthma" patients with a significant psychological component to their symptom presentation.

Given the impressive results of the early work in this area and the striking number of children and adults who suffer from asthma, it behooves clinical hypnosis researchers to undertake further study of the impact of hypnosis training in this population of medical patients. The number of studies demonstrating the strong relationship between panic and asthma and suggestibility and asthma offer a significant promise for the use of hypnosis as an adjunctive resource in pulmonary care. However, the dated literature in this area limits any enthusiasm among medical specialists to include this as a treatment strategy.

Bulimia

While the prevalence of bulimia nervosa in the general population is very small, estimates of women, especially young women, with eating disorders range between 1 and 4 percent (American Psychiatric Association, 2000; Howat & Saxton, 1987). Individuals with this disorder are often normal-weight individuals, but they feel out of control with regard to their eating, often bingeing on large quantities of food at a time. Despite a "normal" appearance, they commonly harbor a distorted body image of themselves as overweight, and they become preoccupied with maintaining a certain physical image. Diuretics and vomiting are often employed to reduce the caloric impact of over-eating that leads to a vicious cycle of bingeing and purging. While these disordered eating behaviors are not life threatening per se, serious dental, gastrointestinal, and cardiovascular problems can result from chronic bingeing and purging (Fairburn, Cooper, Safran, & Wilson, 2008).

The origin of this disorder is unknown, but symptoms of depression and anxiety are frequently reported by those with bulimia. Cognitive-behavioral treatments have been found to be successful at reducing the frequency and severity of bulimic symptoms, although many women report symptoms of this disorder throughout their lives. Dissociative symptoms of timelessness, depersonalization, derealization, and involuntariness have been linked to experiences of bingeing and purging (Demitrack, Putnam, Brewerton, Brandt, & Gold, 1990).

Cognitive-behavioral treatments address several aspects of the symptom picture in bulimia: cognitive restructuring techniques are directed at the patient's body image distortions and irrational ideas regarding food; behavioral strategies are employed to reduce bingeing and purging as well as for affect management. In most cases, clinicians ask patients to keep a record of thoughts and feelings, especially those that occur prior to a binge episode. A review of the errors of logic associated with patients' thinking about body image, food, and nutrition often leads to the revelation of core beliefs that can be revised with more adaptive ideas substituted. Behavioral strategies for relaxation, affect management, and more adaptive eating behaviors are rehearsed in the clinical setting and applied in daily life.

Recent years have seen a number of empirical studies regarding the efficacy of CBT interventions in bulimia. Keel & Haedt (2008) provide a summary of evidence-based studies in this area. Their review supports CBT as a well-established intervention for adults and older adolescents with bulimia nervosa. Randomized controlled trials find better outcomes correlating with patients' advancing age with few successful studies including children and very young adults. Follow-up studies with adolescents and adults in this review showed improvement at six months and one year with symptom and social gains lasting as long as 10 years (Fairburn, Jones, Peveler, Hope, & O'Connor, 1993; Keel, Crow, Davis, & Mitchell, 2002). Support was found for family, interpersonal, and psychodynamic treatments aimed at self-confidence and self-efficacy, offering promise for a more diverse approach to treatment and potential lines of experimental inquiry.

Early reports of dissociative symptoms among this population (Demitrack et al., 1990; Torem, 1986) prompted hypnosis researchers to study the levels of hypnotizability among bulimics. First among these studies were Pettinatti, Horne, and Staats (1985) who found that bulimic inpatients showed elevated scores on hypnotizability scales when compared to anorexic inpatients. College outpatients displayed similar scores on a variety of hypnotizability measures in several reports (Barabasz, 1993; Groth-Marnat & Schumaker, 1990; Kranhold, Baumann, & Fichter, 1992). Young women with bulimia and another group of normal-weight controls who volunteered for an investigation of taste preference were tested for hypnotizability by the same investigator who was blind to diagnosis (Covino, Jimerson, Wolfe, Franko, & Frankel, 1994). Bulimic subjects not only had higher scores than the controls, but an unusual number of these individuals (p < .001) scored in the "highly hypnotizable" range.

Despite good evidence of hypnotizability of bulimic patients with various levels of the disorder, psychological interventions utilizing hypnosis in this population are rare. The few studies that do exist lack appropriate controls, employ small sample sizes, and fail to report follow-up data (Griffiths, Gillett, & Davies, 1989; Vanderlinden & Vandereycken, 1988). Such limitations make it difficult to be confident about advocating for the use of hypnosis with these patients. One controlled study (Griffiths, Hadzi-Pavlovic, & Channon-Little, 1996) randomly assigned subjects to a CBT group or one employing "hypnobehavioral" treatment (HBT). Participants received individual psychotherapy along with manualized care that delivered traditional CBT and HBT to the relevant group. HBT subjects received suggestions for behavioral change and self-hypnosis training with ego-strengthening techniques. Both treatment conditions showed equal effect at nine-month follow-up, but they followed an initial period of behavioral treatment that might have been the efficacious element of the care. A recent study reported by Barabasz (2007) found 14 bulimic women who were randomly assigned to a CBT or CBT + hypnosis group then followed for three months. Symptom measures found comparable results for both treatments, but the hypnosis group reported significantly less binge frequency compared to those treated with CBT alone. While encouraging, this is a very small sample and this study is a singular example of the kind of research that is needed in this area.

Research findings of elevated hypnotizability in this population invite us to believe that hypnosis strategies added to the well-supported CBT interventions for bulimia should make an important addition to medical and psychological care in this area. Patients who are more suggestible should be able to use trance and new ideas to assist them with managing emotions, changing fixed ideas about nutrition and body image, revising maladaptive core beliefs, and practicing more adaptive eating behaviors. The paucity of recent, controlled intervention studies at this point makes it impossible for any provider to be enthusiastic about the use of hypnosis for bulimia. Such work is clearly needed.

Hyperemesis

Uncontrolled nausea and vomiting, also known as hyperemesis, is a common consequence of chemotherapy for cancer and, as we know, of pregnancy. Anticipatory nausea and vomiting (ANV) usually results from the combination of behavioral conditioning and the application of intensive medication regimens that are aimed at reducing cancerous cells (Morrow & Dobkin, 1988). ANV affects between 25 and 50 percent of patients, commonly by the fourth session of treatment (Andrykowski, Redd, & Hatfield, 1985; Redd & Andrykowski, 1982), with patients experiencing symptoms of nausea and vomiting in response to hospital odors, images, or personnel or other conditioned stimuli, and their symptoms are escalated by anxiety (Andrykowski, 1987; Jacobsen, Bovbjerg, & Redd, 1993). ANV is a debilitating experience for patients, but it is, also, the most common reason that cancer patients discontinue treatment earlier than advised (Dolgin, Katz, Doctors, & Siegel, 1986; Sitzia & Huggins, 1998; Zeltzer & LeBaron, 1982). While most women experience nausea and vomiting in the early months of pregnancy, a certain number (0.5–2 percent) experience intractable vomiting leading to dehydration. This condition is called hyperemesis gravidarum (HG), and it results from metabolic changes created by the placenta. Behavioral conditioning can complicate this condition, as with ANV, but psychological factors have not been found to play an etiological role in this condition.

Behavioral intervention procedures are the most widely offered psychosocial services at comprehensive cancer centers due to their immediate impact on the presenting complaint, the relative ease of application and the opportunity to offer some measure of control to a disempowered patient (Coluzzi et al., 1995; Meyer & Mark, 1995). Behavioral interventions typically include distraction techniques such as story telling and the use of video games, systematic desensitization, relaxation training, and hypnosis. In their review of 54 published studies of the effectiveness of interventions aimed at the aversive symptoms of cancer treatments, Redd, Montgomery, & DuHamel (2001) report that behavioral techniques can effectively control anticipatory nausea and vomiting along with anxiety and distress related to the medical treatments. Patients treated with relaxation are able to use this skill during aversive procedures to manage accompanying anxiety and to distract themselves from the subjective experience of nausea. Numerous studies find relaxation to be effective at decreasing the incidence of nausea and vomiting prior to chemotherapy (Razavi et al., 1993; Vasterling, Jenkins, Tope, & Burish, 1993).

Hypnosis has been employed by pediatric and adult clinicians to manage pain, reduce anxiety, and manage the symptoms of nausea and vomiting. Zeltzer, Dolgin, LeBaron, & LeBaron (1991) treated 54 children who were randomly assigned to receive hypnosis, distraction, or placebo interventions. Observation and interview measures of anticipatory- and post-chemotherapy nausea and vomiting, distress, and functional disruption found that children in the hypnosis group had the greatest reduction in symptoms. Another study with children found that hypnosis decreased the need for antiemetic medicines and reduced chemotherapy-related nausea and vomiting (Jacknow, Tschann, Link, & Boyce, 1994). Furthermore, children in the hypnosis group were still able to manage anticipatory nausea for several months after treatment. Among adults, bone marrow transplant patients who were randomly assigned to groups utilizing hypnosis, CBT, therapist contact, and treatment as usual demonstrated better results with hypnosis than with CBT (Syrjala, Cummings, & Donaldson, 1992). In a related use of hypnosis to manage postoperative nausea and vomiting, patients undergoing breast surgery with hypnosis training four to six days prior demonstrated less vomiting and less need for analgesic medications (Enquist, Bjorklund, Engman, & Jakobsson, 1997).

While there is both logic and some empirical support for the use of hypnosis in the management of hyperemesis, especially with regard to ANV among cancer patients, and, perhaps, surgical patients, this literature is dated, the sample sizes are small, and the studies are very few in number. Research combining hypnosis training for distraction, absorption, and anxiety management along with the use of imagined approaches to noxious stimuli in the manner of systematic desensitization holds a great deal of promise for the field and for patient care.

PAROCHIAL RESEARCH: FUNCTIONAL GASTROINTESTINAL DISORDERS AND SMOKING CESSATION

Functional Gastrointestinal Disorders

By definition, the bloating, abdominal pain, and changes in motility and bowel movement that constitute functional gastrointestinal disorders (FGID) are without structural or organic origin (Toner & Cassati, 2002). Disorders such as irritable bowel syndrome (IBS) and functional bowel disorder (FBD) impact as many as 22 percent of the population and comprise close to one-third of the typical gastroenterologist's practice (Drossman, Camilleri, Mayer, & Whitehead, 2002; Whitehead, Crowell, Robinson, Heller, & Schuster, 1992). As with insomnia, autonomic hyperarousal, cognition, and behavior play key roles in maintaining these disorders. In response to experimental stressors, patients with FGID show increased gastric motility (Drossman et al., 2002; Maunder et al., 1997) gastric velocity, and gastric activity (Bilhartz and Croft, 2000; Drossman, Whitehead, & Camilleri 1997). However, dismotility is absent during sleep (Fukudo et al., 1992; Kellow, Gill, & Wingate, 1990). FGID patients selectively attend to abdominal sensations and maintain a persistent belief that they are seriously ill, despite medical assurance to the contrary. Psychological factors such as a history of early childhood abuse and chronic mood disorders are common precursors, with a majority of FGID patients failing to see a mind-body dimension to their disorder (Blanchard, 2001; Toner & Casati, 2002).

While controlled studies utilizing brief psychodynamic psychotherapy have demonstrated success in reducing FGID symptoms (Guthrie, Creed, Dawson, & Tomenson, 1991), substantial research supports the efficacy of cognitive-behavioral interventions for this population (Blanchard, 2000). Techniques including psychophysiological education, relaxation training, cognitive restructuring, and behavioral rehearsal have improved FGID in randomized controlled studies involving waitlist (Tkachuk, Graff, Martin, & Bernstein, 2003; van Dulman, Fennis, & Bleijenberg, 1996) and crossover (Lynch and Zamble, 1989) designs. Treatment strategies that help FGID patients to correct a tendency toward catastrophic thinking, while acquiring adaptive habits such as relaxation, are accepted interventions by mental health and medical caregivers.

Whorwell and his colleagues found that as few as seven 30-minute sessions with hypnosis were effective in reducing IBS symptoms and were more effective than talking therapy alone (Whorwell, Prior, & Faragher, 1984; Whorwell, Prior, & Colgan, 1987; Prior, Colgan, & Whorwell, 1990). Subsequent work from the same group found substantial improvement in pain control, bowel movement, and rectal sensitivity (Houghton, Jackson, Whorwell, & Cooper, 1999) and that bowel symptoms and quality of life remained improved at three months (Gonsalkorale, Houghton, & Whorwell, 2002) and, even, five years (Gonsalkorale, Perrey, Pravica, Whorwell, & Hutchinson, 2003). Similar symptom amelioration and improved quality of life were effected by hypnosis through audiotapes with gains remaining at 10–12 months (Palsson, Turner, Johnson, Burnett, & Whitehead, 2002).

Unfortunately, rather than integrate the significant body of psychological research that finds support for cognitive-behavioral interventions, hypnotic research methods, almost universally, employ the strategy of the earliest hypnosis investigators in this area who specify "gut-directed" suggestions as the desired hypnosis intervention. This recommendation is supported by their observation that six study subjects had prior, general, hypnotic suggestions without relief and these improved when suggestions for warm hands that could soothe the abdomen and bring better control to bowel function were presented to them (Gonsalkorale, 2006; Whorwell et al., 1987). Generalized from such a small and briefly analyzed sample, this logic is not only not com-pelling, it ignores a substantial body of CBT research with its focus on alter-ing cognitions and changing behavior. Only very recently have investigators begun to integrate CBT strategies into hypnosis studies (Taylor, Read, & Hills, 2004), although maintaining the overly specific approach. Such a re-stricted strategy unnecessarily limits the range of therapeutic interventions for patients with FGID and keeps clinicians and investigators, who are involved in similar work, unnecessarily sequestered. Moreover, such an idio-syncratic logic and clinical approach contributes to the marginalization of our field by mental health professionals who witness the ignorance of an evidence-based approach with CBT and by medical practitioners who think it unconventional.

While there is some enthusiasm for the use of hypnosis in this area, randomized control studies and a better integration of the successful ele-ments of CBT research with this patient population are much needed.

Smoking Cessation

Cigarette smoking is responsible for 30 percent of cancer deaths in this country and it is a major contributor to emphysema, heart disease, and stroke, along with presenting a significant health risk for nonsmokers who are exposed to it. Despite significant public education efforts across recent years, the population of smokers in this country remains relatively constant at more than 23 percent (CDC, 2006). Unfortunately, psychological factors of condi-tioning and suggestion combine with the addictive drug nicotine to create a complex habit disorder that undermines most smokers' best intentions.

The elements of "suggestion" are well employed by the tobacco marketers who place attractive people in appealing settings to sell their product. Con-sumers are invited to become imaginatively involved in the advertisement and open to the suggestion that a particularly disagreeable behavior is as de-sirable as the images. Catchy phrases are so repetitiously presented that, many years later, the general public of a certain age knows what LSMFT means, how good Winstons taste, and how cool Joe Camel is. By contrast, public health messages that employ cancerous lungs, a dyspneic cowboy, and illness warnings fail to invite smokers to linger long enough on the content of the commercial to absorb the message. While the numbers are small, about 2 percent of patients will stop when their primary care doctor suggests it to them (Law & Tang, 1995).

The treatment of cigarette smokers has been quite challenging. Most interventions, be they with nicotine replacement, antidepressants, or CBT, are likely to succeed with only one of five patients. However, given the number of smokers and the known consequences of long-term use, these numbers represent a significant health care gain. Research finds support for behavioral techniques such as rapid smoking, stimulus control, and skill training, but not for aversive stimuli, contingency, and nicotine fading (Covino & Bottari, 2001). Given the important role that nicotine plays in fostering and maintaining addiction, it is not surprising to find nicotine replacement almost doubles the chances of success for those who are interested in quitting, regardless of the treatment approach used (Silagy, Lancaster, Stead, Mant, & Fowler, 2004). Most reports on the use of hypnosis for cigarette smoking follow the direct suggestion/motivational model developed by H. Spiegel (1970). This method exhorts patients to know that "smoking is a poison for your body; you need your body to live; and to the extent that you want to live, you owe your body respect and protection." Some investigators use hypnosis to achieve relaxation, to focus on individual motivations to change, and to rehearse coping behaviors.

A popular, although controversial, theory in habit change work is the "transtheoretical" Stages of Change model of Prochaska and his colleagues (Prochaska & Velicer, 1997). This model posits a process of six stages that patients with habit disorders such as cigarette smoking are likely to pass through: precontemplation, contemplation, preparation, action, maintenance, and termination. While there is some caution about the success of this model (Hughes, 2000; Riemsma, Pattenden, Bridle et al., 2002), proponents believe that tailoring suggestions and behavioral recommendations to meet the motivational level and needs of the person undertaking to change behavior will improve treatment outcome for this population (Prochaska, Velicer, Fava et al., 2001).

The hypnosis literature on smoking cessation is a diverse one with a large number of clinical reports dating back to the 1970s. Several quasi-experimental designs with small, unequal, or incomparable samples and questionably reliable outcome measures, and only three studies that meet the criteria for evidence-based treatment comprise most of the body of work in this area (Green & Lynn, 2000). Reviewers point to methodological weaknesses like incomplete descriptions of the "hypnosis intervention," inadequate controls, and an excessive dependence upon unreliable measures of abstinence to assess treatment outcomes (Abbot, Stead, White et al., 1998; Covino & Bottari, 2001; Greene & Lynn, 2000; Law & Tang, 1995). The Cochrane Review assessed nine randomized, controlled studies from 1977 to 1988 and found insufficient evidence to recommend hypnosis; they proposed nonspecific therapist variables as the most likely contributors to treatment success (Abbot, Stead, White, & Barnes, 1998). In a larger review, similar methodological weaknesses were noted, along with the challenge of differentiating the cognitive-behavioral interventional elements from those of hypnosis, but the authors saw hypnotic interventions as superior to various no-treatment conditions (Green & Lynn, 2000). A meta-analysis of 48 investigations found mean quit-rates of 36 percent with hypnosis as superior to physician advice at 2 percent (Viswesvaran and Schmidt, 1992). Most conclude that the use of hypnosis for smoking cessation is better than no treatment, but it cannot be seen as superior, except to placebo, aversive conditioning, and physician advice.

The use of hypnosis for smoking cessation is among the best examples of what contributes to the marginalization of this technique. On the one hand, research substantiates that it could be effective, and, indeed, that it is more effective than no treatment at all. Thus, it is worth the work to update and to make more sophisticated the research methodologies in this area. However, by largely ignoring the strong evidence in support of nicotine replacement, failing to integrate the compatible behavioral techniques that work and to explore the potential assistance that the transtheoretical model offers, hypnosis researchers make it very difficult for colleagues to take our work seriously and to include it as a component of treatment.

CONCLUSIONS

For many years, hypnosis-trained clinicians have advocated to a largely unreceptive audience of medical practitioners that they had something to offer their patients. The best work in this field has established a clear role for hypnosis in the treatment of patients with pain (Patterson & Jensen, 2003). Surgical interventions and procedures offer the similar opportunity to address the complex interactions of anxiety, pain, treatment time, and patient compliance with adjunctive hypnotic strategies. There is, as has been shown, some real promise for the use of hypnosis with many medical illnesses and conditions. For this technique to be better accepted, it is imperative that researchers in the field update outdated studies, integrate promising strategies from related research, abandon idiosyncrasy, bring appropriate scientific rigor to investigations, and pay attention to the excellent work of colleagues in related fields. With enthusiasm for this approach, it is clear that patients will benefit from our skills and the field will be brought closer to mainstream practice.

REFERENCES

Abbot, N. C., Stead, L. F., White, A. R., Barnes, J., & Ernst, E. (2000). Hypnotherapy for smoking cessation. *Cochrane Database of Systematic Reviews, 2,* CD001008.

Alexander, F. & French, T.M. (1948). *Studies in psychosomatic medicine.* New York: Ronald Press.

American Psychiatric Association Work Group on Eating Disorders. Practice guideline for the treatment of patients with eating disorders (revision). *American Journal of Psychiatry, 157*(1), 1–39.

Anbar, R.D. (2002). Hypnosis in pediatrics: Applications at a pediatric pulmonary center. *BMC Pediatrics, 3,* 2–11.

Anderson, N. B., & Elizabeth, N. B. (2003). *Emotional longevity: What really determines how long you live.* New York: Viking Press.

Andrykowski, M. A. (1987). Do infusion-related tastes and odors facilitate the development of anticipatory nausea? A failure to support hypothesis. *Health Psychology, 6*(4), 329–341.

Andrykowski, M. A., Redd, W. H., & Hatfield, A. K. (1985). Development of anticipatory nausea: A prospective analysis. *Journal of Consulting and Clinical Psychology, 53*(4), 447–454.

Barabasz, M. (1990). Treatment of bulimia with hypnosis involving awareness and control in clients with high dissociative capacity. *Journal of Psychosomatic Research, 37*(1–4), 53–56.

Barabasz, M. (2007). Efficacy of hypnotherapy in the treatment of eating disorders. *International Journal of Clinical and Experimental Hypnosis, 55*(3), 318–335.

Bastien, C. H., Morin, C. M., Ouellet, M. C., Blais, F. C., & Bouchard, S. (2004). Cognitive-behavioral therapy for insomnia: Comparison of individual therapy, group therapy, and telephone consultations. *Journal of Consulting and Clinical Psychology, 72*(4), 653–659.

Ben-Zvi, Z., Spohn, W. A., Young, S. H., & Kattan, M. (1982). Hypnosis for exercise-induced asthma. *American Review of Respiratory Disease, 125*(4), 392–395.

Bilhartz, L. E. & Croft, C. L. (2000). *Gastrointestinal disease in primary care.* Philadelphia: Lippincott, Williams, & Wilkins.

Blanchard, E. B. (2001). *Irritable bowel syndrome: Psychosocial assessment and treatment.* Washington, DC: American Psychological Association.

Bonnet, M. H. & Arand, D. L. (1998). Heart rate variability in insomniacs and matched normal sleepers. *Psychosomatic Medicine, 60*(5), 610–615.

Bonnet, M. H., & Arand, D. L. (2003). Insomnia, metabolic rate and sleep restoration. *Journal of Internal Medicine, 254*(1), 23–31.

British Tuberculosis Association. (1968). Hypnosis for asthma: A controlled trial. *British Medical Journal, 4*(5623), 71–76.

Butler, L. D., Symons, B. K., Henderson, S. L., Shortliffe, L. D., & Spiegel, D. (2005). Hypnosis reduces distress and duration of an invasive medical procedure for children. *Pediatrics, 115*(1), 77–85.

Centers for Disease Control and Prevention. (2006). Cigarette smoking among adults. *Morbidity and Mortality Weekly Report, 56*(44), 1157–1161.

Christen, A. G. (2001). Tobacco cessation, the dental profession, and the role of dental education. *Journal of Dental Education, 65*(4), 368–374.

Coluzzi, P. H., Grant, M., Doroshow, J. H., Rhiner, M., Ferrell, B., & Rivera, L. (1995). Survey of the provision of supportive care services at National Cancer Institute-designated cancer centers. *Journal of Clinical Oncology, 13,* 756–764.

Covino, N.A. (2008). Medical illnesses, conditions and procedures. (Chapter 25) In M. R. Nash & A. Barnier (Eds.), *The Oxford handbook of hypnosis: Theory, research and practice.* Oxford, U.K.: Oxford University Press.

Covino, N.A., & Bottari, M. (2001). Hypnosis, behavioral theory and smoking cessation. *Journal of Dental Education, 65,* 340–347.

Covino, N. A., Jimerson, D. C., Wolfe, B. E., Franko, D. L., & Frankel, F. H. (1994). Hypnotizability, dissociation, and bulimia nervosa. *Journal of Abnormal Psychology, 103*(3), 455–459.

Demitrack, M. A., Putnam, F. W., Brewerton, T. D., Brandt, H. A., & Gold, P. W. (1990). Relation of clinical variables to dissociative phenomena in eating disorders. *American Journal of Psychiatry, 147*(9), 1184–1188.

Dolgin, M. J., Katz, E. R., Doctors, S. R., & Siegel, S. E. (1986). Caregivers' perceptions of medical compliance in adolescents with cancer. *Journal of Adolescent Health, 7*(1), 22–27.

Drossman, D. A., Camilleri, M., Mayer, E. A., & Whitehead, W. E. (2002). AGA technical review on irritable bowel syndrome. *Gastroenterology, 123*(6), 2108–2131.

Drossman, D. A., Whitehead, W. E., & Camilleri, M. (1997). Irritable bowel syndrome: A technical review for practice guideline development. *Gastroenterology, 112*(6), 2120–2037.

Edinger, J. D., Olsen, M. K., Stechuchak, K. M., Means, M. K., Lineberger, M. D., Kirby, A., et al. (2009). Cognitive behavioral therapy for patients with primary insomnia or insomnia associated predominantly with mixed psychiatric disorders: A randomized clinical trial. *Sleep, 32*(4), 499–510.

Enqvist, B., Björklund, C., Engman, M., & Jakobsson, J. (1997). Preoperative hypnosis reduces postoperative vomiting after surgery of the breasts. A prospective, randomized and blinded study. *Acta Anaesthesiologica Scandinavica, 41*(8), 1028–1032.

Ewer, T. C., & Stewart, D. E. (1986). Improvement in bronchial hyper-responsiveness in patients with moderate asthma after treatment with a hypnotic technique: A randomised controlled trial. *British Medical Journal (Clin Res Ed), 293*(6555), 1129–1132.

Fairburn, C. G., Cooper, Z., Shafran, R., & Wilson, G. T. (2008). *Eating disorders: A transdiagnostic protocol.* In D. Barlow (Ed.), *Clinical handbook of psychological disorders: A step-by-step treatment manual.* New York: Guilford Press.

Fairburn, C. G., Jones, R., Peveler, R. C., Hope, R. A., & O'Connor, M. (1993). Psychotherapy and bulimia nervosa. Longer-term effects of interpersonal psychotherapy, behavior therapy, and cognitive behavior therapy. *Archives of General Psychiatry, 50*(6), 419–428.

Foley, D. J., Monjan, A. A., Brown, S. L., Simonsick, E. M., Wallace, R. B., & Blazer, D. G. (1995). Sleep complaints among elderly persons: An epidemiologic study of three communities. *Sleep, 18*(6), 425–432.

French, T. M. & Alexander, F. (1941). Psychogenic factors in bronchial asthma, part II. *Psychoanalytic Review, 30*, 109–110.

Fukudo, S., Muranaka, M., Nomura, T., & Satake, M. (1992). Brain-gut interactions in irritable bowel syndrome: Physiological and psychological aspect. *Nippon Rinsho, 50*(11), 2703–2711.

Giardino, N. D., McGrady, A., & Andrasik, F. (2007). Relaxation therapies for somatic disorders. In P. M. Lehrer, R. L. Woolfolk, & W. F. Sime (Eds.), *Principles and practice of stress management.* New York: Guilford Press.

Gonsalkorale, W. M. (2006). Gut-directed hypnotherapy: The Manchester approach for treatment of irritable bowel syndrome. *International Journal of Clinical and Experimental Hypnosis, 54*(1), 27–50.

Gonsalkorale, W. M., Houghton, L. A., & Whorwell, P. J. (2002). Hypnotherapy in irritable bowel syndrome: A large-scale audit of a clinical service with examination of factors influencing responsiveness. *American Journal of Gastroenterology, 97*(4), 954–961.

Gonsalkorale, W. M., Perrey, C., Pravica, V., Whorwell, P. J., & Hutchinson, I. V. (2003). Interleukin 10 genotypes in irritable bowel syndrome: Evidence for an inflammatory component? *Gut, 52*(1), 91–93.

Goodwin, T. M. (2008). Hyperemesis gravidarum. *Obstetrics & Gynecology Clinics of North America, 35*(3), 401–417.

Green, J. P., & Lynn, S. J. (2000). Hypnosis and suggestion-based approaches to smoking cessation. *International Journal of Clinical and Experimental Hypnosis, 48*(2), 195–223.

Griffiths, M. D., Gillett, C. A., & Davies, P. (1989). Hypnotic suppression of conditioned electrodermal responses. *Perceptual & Motor Skills, 69*(1), 186.

Griffiths, R. A., Hadzi-Pavlovic, D., & Channon-Little, L. (1996). The short-term follow-up effects of hypnobehavioural and cognitive behavioural treatment for bulimia nervosa. *European Eating Disorders Review, 4*(1), 12–31.

Grossman, P., Niemann, L., Schmidt, S., & Walach, H. (2004). Mindfulness-based stress reduction and health benefits: A meta-analysis. *Journal of Psychosomatic Research, 57*(1), 35–43.

Groth-Marnat, G., & Schumaker, J. F. (1990). Hypnotizability, attitudes toward eating, and concern with body size in a female college population. *American Journal of Clinical Hypnosis, 32*(3), 194–200.

Guthrie, E., Creed, F., Dawson, D., & Tomenson, B. (1991). A controlled trial of psychological treatment for the irritable bowel syndrome. *Gastroenterology, 100*(2), 450–457.

Harvey, A. G. (2000). Pre-sleep cognitive activity: A comparison of sleep-onset insomniacs and good sleepers. *British Journal of Clinical Psychology, 39,* 275–286.

Hasler, G., Gergen, P. J., Kleinbaum, D. G., Ajdacic, V., Gamma, A., Eich, D., et al. (2005). Asthma and panic in young adults: A 20-year prospective community study. *American Journal of Respiratory and Critical Care Medicine, 171,* 1224–1230.

Hauri, P. & Linde, S. (1996). *No more sleepless nights.* New York: Wiley.

Hiller, W., Leibbrand, R., Rief, W., & Fichter, M. M. (2002). Predictors of course and outcome in hypochondriasis after cognitive-behavioral treatment. *Psychotherapy and Psychosomatics, 71*(6), 318–325.

Houghton, L. A., Jackson, N. A., Whorwell, P. J., & Cooper, S. M. (1999). 5-HT4 receptor antagonism in irritable bowel syndrome: Effect of SB-207266-A on rectal sensitivity and small bowel transit. *Alimentary Pharmacology & Therapeutics, 13*(11), 1437–1444.

Howat, P. M. & Saxton, A. M. (1988). The incidence of bulimic behavior in a secondary and university school population. *Journal of Youth and Adolescence, 17*(3).

Hughes, J. R. (2000). New treatments for smoking cessation. *California Journal for Clinicians,* 50:140–142.

Jacknow, D. S., Tschann, J. M., Link, M. P., & Boyce, W. T. (1994). Hypnosis in the prevention of chemotherapy-related nausea and vomiting in children: A prospective study. *Journal of Developmental & Behavioral Pediatrics, 15*(4), 258–264.

Jacobs, G. D., Pace-Schott, E. F., Stickgold, R., & Otto, M. W. (2004). Cognitive behavior therapy and pharmacotherapy for insomnia: A randomized controlled trial and direct comparison. *Archives of Internal Medicine, 164*(17), 1888–1896.

Jacobsen, P. B., Bovbjerg, D. H., & Redd, W. H. (1993). Anticipatory anxiety in women receiving chemotherapy for breast cancer. *Health Psychology, 12*(6), 469–475.

Jones, N. F., Kinsman, R. A., Dirks, J. F., & Dahlem, N. W. (1979). Psychological contributions to chronicity in asthma: Patient response styles influencing medical treatment and its outcome. *Medical Care, 17*(11), 1103–1118.

Katon, W. J., Richardson, L., Lozano, P., & McCauley, E. (2004). The relationship of asthma and anxiety disorders. *Psychosomatic Medicine, 66*(3), 349–355.

Keel, P. K., Crow, S., Davis, T. L., & Mitchell, J. E. (2002). Assessment of eating disorders: Comparison of interview and questionnaire data from a long-term follow-up study of bulimia nervosa. *Journal of Psychosomatic Research, 53,* 1043–1047.

Keel, P. K., & Haedt, A. (2008). Evidence-based psychosocial treatments for eating problems and eating disorders. *Journal of Clinical Child & Adolescent Psychology, 37*(1), 39–61.

Kellow, J. E., Gill, R. C., & Wingate, D. L. (1990). Prolonged ambulant recordings of small bowel motility demonstrate abnormalities in the irritable bowel syndrome. *Gastroenterology, 98*(5), 1208–1218.

Kinsman, R. A., Dirks, J. F., Jones, N. F., Dahlem, N. W. (1980). Anxiety reduction in asthma: four catches to general application. *Psychosomatic Medicine, 42*(4), 397–405.

Kranhold, C., Baumann, U., & Fichter, M. (1992). Hypnotizability in bulimic patients and controls. A pilot study. *European Archives of Psychiatry and Clinical Neuroscience, 242*(2-3), 72–76.

Kuisk, L. A., Bertelson, A. D., & Walsh, J. K. (1989). Presleep cognitive hyperarousal and affect as factors in objective and subjective insomnia. *Perceptual & Motor Skills, 69*(3), 1219–1225.

Lang, E. V., Benotsch, E. G., Fick, L. J., Lutgendorf, S., Berbaum, M. L., Berbaum, K. S.,(2000). Adjunctive nonpharmacological analgesia for invasive medical procedures:a randomised trial. *Lancet, (355),* 1486–90.

Law M., & Tang J. L. (1997). An analysis of the effectiveness of interventions intended to help people stop smoking. *Archives of Internal Medicine, (337),* 1195–202.

Lehrer, P. M., Carr, R., Sargunaraj, D., & Woolfolk, R. L. (1994). Stress management techniques: Are they all equivalent, or do they have specific effects? *Biofeedback & Self Regulation, 19*(4), 353–401.

Logan, H., & Spiegel, D. (2000). Adjunctive non-pharmacological analgesia for invasive medical procedures: A randomised trial. *Lancet, 355*(9214), 1486–1490.

Luparello, T., Lyons, H. A., Bleecker, E. R., & McFadden Jr., E. R. (1968). Influences of suggestion on airway reactivity in asthmatic subjects. *Psychosomatic Medicine, 30*(6), 819–825.

Lushington, K., Dawson, D., & Lack, L. (2000). Core body temperature is elevated during constant wakefulness in aged poor sleepers. *Sleep, 4,* 1–5.

Lyles, J. N., Burish, T. G., Krozely, M. G., & Oldham, R. K. (1982). Efficacy of relaxation training and guided imagery in reducing the aversiveness of cancer chemotherapy. *Journal of Consulting and Clinical Psychology, 50*(4), 509–524.

Lynch, P. M. & Zamble, E. (1989). A controlled behavioural treatment study of irritable bowel syndrome. *Behavioral Therapy, 20*, 509–523.

Maher-Loughnan, G. P., Mason, A. A., Macdonald, N., & Fry, L. (1962). Controlled trial of hypnosis in the symptomatic treatment of asthma. *British Medical Journal, 2*(5301), 371–376.

Maunder, R. G., de Rooy, E. C., Toner, B. B., Greenberg, G. R., Steinhart, A. H., McLeod, R. S., et al. (1997). Health-related concerns of people who receive psychological support for inflammatory bowel disease. *Canadian Journal of Gastroenterology, 111*(8), 681–685.

Mendoza, M. E., Capafons, A., Espejo, B., & Montalvo, D. (2009). Beliefs and attitudes toward hypnosis of Spanish psychologists. *Psicothema, 21*(3), 465–470.

Meyer, T. J., & Mark, M. M. (1995). Effects of psychosocial interventions with adult cancer patients: A meta-analysis of randomized experiments. *Health Psychology, 14*(2), 99–101.

Montgomery, G. H., DuHamel, K. N., & Redd, W. H. (2000). A meta-analysis of hypnotically induced analgesia: How effective is hypnosis? *International Journal of Clinical and Experimental Hypnosis, 48*, 138–153.

Morin, C. M., Colecchi, C., Stone, J., Sood, R., & Brink, D. (1999). Behavioral and pharmacological therapies for late-life insomnia: A randomized controlled trial. *Journal of the American Medical Association, 281*, 991–999.

Morrow, G. R. & Dobkin, P. L. (1987). Behavioral approaches for the management of adversive side effects of cancer treatment. *Psychiatric Medicine, 5*(4), 299–314.

Morrow, G. R. & Dobkin, P. (1988). Behavioural factors influencing the development and expression of chemotherapy induced side effects. *British Journal of Cancer, 66*(XIX), 54–61.

National Heart Lung and Blood Institute. (2008). What is asthma? *Diseases and Conditions Index.* Retrieved from http://www.nhlbi.nih.gov/health/dci/Diseases/Asthma/Asthma_WhatIs.html.

National Heart, Lung, and Blood Institute. (1998). *Insomnia: Assessment and management in primary care* (NIH Pub. No. 98-4088). Bethesda, MD: NHLBI.

National Institutes of Health (1998). Insomnia: Assessment and Management in Primary Care. US Department of Health and Human Services; National Heart, Lung and Blood Institute. NIH Publication No. 98-4088.

National Institutes of Health. (2005). *State-of-the-Science Conference Statement.* Bethesda, MD: August 18, 2005.

Nelson, J., & Harvey, A. G. (2003). An exploration of pre-sleep cognitive activity in insomnia: Imagery and verbal thought. *British Journal of Clinical Psychology, 42*(3), 271–288.

Palsson, O. S., Turner, M. J., Johnson, D. A., Burnett, C. K., & Whitehead, W. E. (2002). Hypnosis treatment for severe irritable bowel syndrome: investigation of mechanism and effects on symptoms. *Digestive Diseases and Sciences, 47*(11), 2605–2614.

Patterson, D. R., & Jensen, M. (2003). Hypnosis and clinical pain control. *Psychological Bulletin, 129*(4), 495–521.

Pettinati, H. M., Horne, R. L., & Staats, J. M. (1985). Hypnotizability in patients with anorexia nervosa and bulimia. *Archives of General Psychiatry, 42*(10), 1014–1016.

Pinnell, C. M. & Covino, N. A. (2000). Empirical findings on the use of hypnosis in medicine: A critical review. *International Journal of Clinical and Experimental Hypnosis, 48*(2), 170–194.

Prior, A., Colgan, S. M., & Whorwell, P. J. (1990). Changes in rectal sensitivity after hypnotherapy in patients with irritable bowel syndrome. *Gut, 31*(8), 896–898.

Prochaska, J. O., & Velicer, W. F. (1997). The transtheoretical model of health behavior change. *American Journal of Health Promotion, 12*(1), 38–48.

Prochaska, J. O., Velicer, W. F., Fava, J. L., Rossi, J. S., & Tsoh, J. Y. (2001). Evaluating a population-based recruitment approach and a stage-based expert system intervention for smoking cessation. *Addictive Behaviors, 26*, 583–602.

Razavi, D., Delvaux, N., Farvacques, C., De Brier, F., Van Heer, C., Kaufman, L., et al. (1993). Prevention of adjustment disorders and anticipatory nausea secondary to adjuvant chemotherapy: A double-blind, placebo-controlled study assessing the usefulness of alprazolam. *Journal of Clinical Oncology, 11*(7), 1384–1390.

Redd, W. H. & Andrykowski, M. A. (1982). Behavioral intervention in cancer treatment: Controlling aversion reactions to chemotherapy. *Journal of Consulting and Clinical Psychology, 50*(6), 1018–1029.

Redd, W. H., Montgomery, G. H., & DuHamel, K. N. (2001). Behavioral intervention for cancer treatment side effects. *Journal of the National Cancer Institute, 93*(11), 810–823.

Riemsma, R.P., Pattenden, J, Bridle, C., Sowden, A.J., Mather, L., Watt, I.S., & Walker, A. (2003). Systematic review of the effectiveness of stage based interventions to promote smoking cessation. *BMJ (British Medical Journal), 327* (7400), 1175–1177.

Roy-Byrne, P., Davidson, K., Kessler, R. C., Amundson, G., Goodwin, R., Kubansky, L., et al. (2008). Anxiety disorders and comorbid medical illness. *General Hospital Psychiatry, 30*(3), 208–225.

Scott, K. M., Von Korff, M., Ormel, J., Zhang, M. Y., Bruffaerts, R., Alonso, J., et al. (2007). Mental disorders among adults with asthma: Results from the World Mental Health Survey. *General Hospital Psychiatry, 29*(2), 123–133.

Silagy, C., Lancaster, T., Stead, L., Mant, D., & Fowler, G. (2004). Nicotine replacement therapy for smoking cessation. *Cochrane Database of Systematic Reviews,* Issue 1. Art. No.: CD000146. DOI:10.1002/14651858.CD000146.pub3.

Sitzia, J., & Huggins, L. (1998). Side effects of cyclophosphamide, methotrexate, and 5- fluorouracil (CMF) chemotherapy for breast cancer. *Cancer Practice,* 6(1),13–21.

Spiegel H. (1970). A single treatment method to stop smoking using ancillary self-hypnosis. *International Journal of Clinical and Experimental Hypnosis, 18*, 235–50.

Syrjala, K. L., Cummings, C., & Donaldson, G. W. (1992). Hypnosis or cognitive behavioral training for the reduction of pain and nausea during cancer treatment: A controlled clinical trial. *Pain, 48*(2), 137–146.

Taylor, E. E., Read, N. W., & Hills, H. M. (2004). Combined group cognitive-behaviour therapy and hypnotherapy in the management of the irritable bowel syndrome: The feasibility of clinical provision. *Behavioural and Cognitive Psychotherapy, 32*(1), 99–106.

Tkachuk, G. A., Graff, L. A., Martin, G. L., & Bernstein, C. N. (2003). Randomized controlled trial of cognitive-behavioral group therapy for irritable bowel syndrome in a medical setting. *Journal of Clinical Psychology in Medical Settings, 10*(1), 57–69.

Toner, B. B., & Casati, J. (2002). *Diseases of the digestive system*. In T. J. Boll, S. B. Johnson, N. W. Perry, & R. H. Rozensky (Eds.), *Handbook of clinical health psychology*. Washington, DC: American Psychological Association.

Torem, M. S. (1986). Dissociative states presenting as an eating disorder. *American Journal of Clinical Hypnosis, 29*(2), 137–142.

U.S. Department of Health and Human Services. (2004) *The Health Consequences of Smoking: A Report of the Surgeon General*. Rockville, MD: U.S. Department of Health and Human Services, Centers for Disease Control and Prevention, National Center for Chronic Disease Prevention and Health Promotion, Office on Smoking and Health.

van Dulmen, A.M., Fennis, J. F., & Bleijenberg, G. (1996). Cognitive-behavioral group therapy for irritable bowel syndrome: effects and long-term follow-up. *Psychosomatic Medicine, 58*(5), 508–514.

Vanderlinden, J., & Vandereycken, W. (1988). Perception of changes in eating disorder patients during group treatment. *Psychotherapy and Psychosomatics, 49*(3–4), 160–163.

Vasterling, J., Jenkins, R. A., Tope, D. M., & Burish, T. G. (1993). Cognitive distraction and relaxation training for the control of side effects due to cancer chemotherapy. *Journal of Behavioral Medicine, 16*(1), 65–80.

Viswesvaran, C., & Schmidt, F. L. (1992). A meta-analytic comparison of the effectiveness of smoking cessation methods. *Journal of Applied Psychology, 77*(4), 554–561.

Vollmer, A., & Blanchard, E. B. (1998). Controlled comparison of individual versus group cognitive therapy for irritable bowel syndrome. *Behavior Therapy, 29*(1), 19–33.

Whitehead, W. E., Crowell, M. D., Robinson, J. C., Heller, B. R., & Schuster, M. M. (1992). Effects of stressful life events on bowel symptoms: Subjects with irritable bowel syndrome compared with subjects without bowel dysfunction. *Gut, 33*(6), 825–830.

Whorwell, P. J., Prior, A., & Colgan, S. M. (1987). Hypnotherapy in severe irritable bowel syndrome: further experience. *Gut, 28*(4), 423–425.

Whorwell, P. J., Prior, A., & Faragher, E. B. (1984). Controlled trial of hypnotherapy in the treatment of severe refractory irritable-bowel syndrome. *Lancet, 2*(8414), 1232–1234.

Wright, R. J. (2004). Alternative modalities for asthma that reduce stress and modify mood states: Evidence for underlying psychobiologic mechanisms. *Annals of Allergy, Asthma & Immunology, 93*(2), S18–23.

Yeatts, K., Sly, P., Shore, S., Weiss, S., Martinez, F., Geller, A., et al. (2006). A brief targeted review of susceptibility factors, environmental exposures, asthma incidence, and recommendations for future asthma incidence research. *Environmental Health Perspectives, 114*(4), 634–640.

Zeltzer, L., & LeBaron, S. (1982). Hypnosis and nonhypnotic techniques for reduction of pain and anxiety during painful procedures in children and adolescents with cancer. *Journal of Pediatrics, 101*, 1032–1035.

Zeltzer, L. K., Dolgin, M. J., LeBaron, S., & LeBaron, C. (1991). A randomized, controlled study of behavioral intervention for chemotherapy distress in children with cancer. *Pediatrics, 88*(1), 34–42.

About the Editor and Contributors

THE EDITOR

Deirdre Barrett, PhD, is a psychologist on the faculty of Harvard Medical School's Behavioral Medicine Program. She is the past president of both the International Association for the Study of Dreams and the American Psychological Association's Division 30: Society of Psychological Hypnosis. Dr. Barrett has written four books: *The Committee of Sleep* (Random House, 2001); *The Pregnant Man and Other Cases from a Hypnotherapist's Couch* (Random House, 1998); *Waistland* (Norton, 2007); and *Supernormal Stimuli* (Norton, 2010). She is an editor of two additional books, *The New Science of Dreaming* (Praeger/Greenwood, 2007) and *Trauma and Dreams* (Harvard University Press, 1996), and has published dozens of academic articles and chapters on health, hypnosis, and dreams. She is editor-in-chief of *DREAMING: The Journal of the Association for the Study of Dreams*.

Dr. Barrett's commentary on psychological issues has been featured on *Good Morning America*, *The Today Show*, CNN, Fox, and the Discovery Channel. She has been interviewed for dream articles in the *Washington Post*, the *New York Times*, *Life*, *Time*, and *Newsweek*. Her own articles have appeared in *Psychology Today* and *Invention and Technology*. Dr. Barrett has lectured at Esalen, the Smithsonian, and universities around the world.

THE CONTRIBUTORS

Arreed Franz Barabasz, EdD, PhD, ABPP, completed his first doctoral degree at State University of New York at Albany at the age of 23. His PhD in Clinical and Human Experimental Psychology is from the University of Canterbury, New Zealand, where he conducted the first studies of EEG and hypnosis in Antarctica. His post-doctoral clinical fellowship was at Massachusetts General Hospital and Harvard Medical School. He is the editor of the *International Journal of Clinical and Experimental Hypnosis* (IJCEH) and professor at Washington State University. He is a diplomat of the American Board of Professional Psychology;

a fellow of the American Psychological Association, the American Psychological Society, and the Society for Clinical and Experimental Hypnosis; and past president of the Society for Clinical and Experimental Hypnosis (SCEH) and of APA Division 30: Society of Psychological Hypnosis. Barabasz was an associate professor of psychology at the Harvard Medical School prior to his professorship at Washington State University. He has published over 125 refereed research papers and received numerous awards for his achievements in research, theory, and practice. He is the three-time winner of the Guze Award from SCEH "for best research paper published in the previous year," most recently in 1999 for his experimental research showing unique EEG ERP responses to hypnosis. His (2005) text *Hypnotherapeutic Techniques, 2E*, coauthored with John G. Watkins, was awarded the 2005 Best Book on Hypnosis by the Society for Clinical and Experimental Hypnosis. His latest psychoanalytic text is Watkins & Barabasz (2008, Routledge) *Advanced Hypnotherapy: Psychodynamic Techniques*. His most recent edited book, also from Routledge, *Medical Hypnosis Primer: Clinical and Research Evidence* (2010) has been adopted by both the Society for Clinical and Experimental Hypnosis and the International Society of Hypnosis for distribution to clinics and hospitals worldwide.

Kent Cadegan, BSc, MD, FCFP, is a medical director at the Glace Bay Site, Cape Breton Regional Hospital, Nova Scotia, Canada. He is also a member of the Medical Advisory Committee of the Cape Breton Regional Hospital. Dr. Cadegan has practiced cradle to grave, home and hospital family medicine for over 33 years in his home town of Glace Bay, Cape Breton. He is a past president of the Clinical Hypnosis Society of Nova Scotia, approved consultant ASCH, Private Practice in Family Medicine, Obstetrics and Hypnosis. He is a founding member of the Canadian Federation of Clinical Hypnosis and serves on its executive board He is a lecturer in the Department of Family Medicine, Dalhousie University, Halifax, Nova Scotia. He is an active organizer and teacher of hypnosis workshops.

Nicholas A. Covino is the president of the Massachusetts School of Professional Psychology (MSPP). For twenty years, he was a psychologist at the Beth Israel Hospital and the Harvard Medical School, where he served as director of the psychology division and as the director of training. He is a member of the Boston Psychoanalytic Society and Institute and maintains a small psychotherapy practice. Covino is past president of the Society for Clinical and Experimental Hypnosis and the author of a number of articles and chapters on the application of clinical hypnosis.

Nicole Flory, PhD, is a licensed clinical psychologist with a private practice in Arlington, Massachusetts, and a teaching associate in the behavioral medicine program at Cambridge Health Alliance, Harvard Medical School. Dr. Flory is dedicated to women's health issues and has conducted a randomized controlled trial on the psychosocial outcomes of hysterectomy. Her research, clinical, and training interests are in cognitive-behavioral interventions, sex and couples therapy, and medical hypnosis. She was born and raised in Europe and completed her initial training on the use of hypnotic techniques in 1995 at the University of Berlin (Freie Universitaet) in Germany. Dr. Flory is the former associate director of the Non-Pharmacologic Analgesics Program, Department of Radiology, Beth Israel Deaconess Medical Center, Harvard Medical School, Boston. She has published in a variety of scientific journals. Dr. Flory enjoys teaching, writing articles, and has received numerous rewards for her work such as the Student Research Award from the Society for Sex Therapy & Research; a research grant from the Canadian Foundation for Women's Health; and the Ruth L. Kirschstein National Research Service Award from the National Institutes of Health (NIH) and the National Cancer Institute (NCI).

V. Krishna Kumar is a professor of psychology at West Chester University of Pennsylvania. He is a clinical associate at the Center for Cognitive Therapy, University of Pennsylvania. He is an elected fellow of APA as well as in two APA divisions, Society of Psychological Hypnosis (Division 30) and Society of Humanistic Psychology (Division 32). He is a two-time recipient of the *Milton Erickson Award for Excellence in Scientific Writing on Clinical Hypnosis* from the American Society of Clinical Hypnosis. He is also a recipient of the *Best Theoretical Paper Award* from Division 30 of the American Psychological Association. He is a past president of the Greater Philadelphia Society of Clinical Hypnosis. He is the author or coauthor of over one hundred articles in peer-reviewed journals and several chapters in edited works.

Elvira Lang, MD, FSIR, FSCEH, is a pioneer and leading expert in the use of hypnosis during medical procedures. Her research-based refinement of hypnotic techniques has resulted in greater patient comfort, increased practitioner effectiveness, and improved financial performance. Dr. Lang is associate professor of radiology at Harvard Medical School and founder of Hypnalgesics, LLC, which trains medical teams in rapid rapport and quick hypnotic techniques. She is internationally known in the field of interventional radiology; she served as chief of interventional radiology at Beth Israel Deaconess Medical Center, Harvard School of Medicine, in Boston from 1998 through 2006. Dr. Lang has trained nurses, doctors, and technologists to incorporate procedure hypnosis into medical areas from a variety of disciplines including MRI, breast care, oncology, urology, gastroenterology, diagnostic and interventional radiology, obstetrics, and dentistry. She held faculty appointments and leadership positions at the University of Heidelberg, Stanford University, the University of Iowa Hospital and Clinics, and the Beth Israel Deaconess Medical Center. Dr. Lang takes an active leadership role in the advance of hypnosis in the medical setting; she is past president of the New England Society of Clinical Hypnosis and current president of the Society of Clinical and Experimental Hypnosis. She is author of *Patient Sedation without Medication: Rapid Rapport and Quick Hypnotic Techniques. A Resource Guide for Doctors, Nurses, and Technologists.*

Stephen R. Lankton, MSW, DAHB, is a licensed clinical social worker in Phoenix, Arizona. He is the editor-in-chief of the *American Journal of Clinical Hypnosis* and a fellow and approved consultant of the American Society of Clinical Hypnosis. He serves as secretary and treasurer of the Arizona Behavioral Health Examiners Board Credential Committee. He is a diplomate in clinical hypnosis, and past-president of the American Hypnosis Board for Clinical Social Work; a fellow of the American Association of Marriage and Family Therapy; and a fellow and board member of the American Psychotherapy Association. Among his awards, Lankton is the recipient of the "Lifetime Achievement Award for Outstanding Contribution to the Field of Psychotherapy" from the Milton Erickson Foundation, 1994 and the "Irving Sector Award for the Advancement of Clinical Hypnosis" from the American Society of Clinical Hypnosis, 2007. He is the author of 18 clinical books, with translations in several languages, regarding techniques of hypnosis, family therapy, and brief therapy. He is currently a psychotherapist in private practice in Phoenix and conducts professional training seminars throughout the world.

Kevin Miller is completing his graduate training in psychology at The Massachusetts School of Professional Psychology. Kevin is also a commissioned officer in the U.S. Navy.

Dr. Jessica Wexler is a graduate of the Massachusetts School of Professional Psychology. After several years as a licensed clinician in Israel working within the immigrant community, Dr. Wexler has returned to the US as a psychologist in private practice. She has a general practice of clinical psychology with a specialty in the treatment of anxiety disorders.

Michael D. Yapko, PhD, is a clinical psychologist in Fallbrook, California. He is internationally recognized for his work in advancing clinical hypnosis and outcome-focused psychotherapy, routinely teaching to professional audiences all over the world. Dr. Yapko has had a special interest for more than three decades in the intricacies of brief therapy and the clinical applications of hypnosis and directive methods. He is the author of ten books and editor of three others, as well as numerous book chapters and articles. These include his widely used classic text, *Trancework: An Introduction to the Practice of Clinical Hypnosis* (3rd ed.), the award-winning *Treating Depression with Hypnosis: Integrating Cognitive-Behavioral and Strategic Approaches* (2001), *Hypnosis and Treating Depression: Applications in Clinical Practice* (2006), as well as *Essentials of Hypnosis* and *Hypnosis and the Treatment of Depressions*. He has produced many CD and DVD programs. His works have been translated into nine languages. More information about Dr. Yapko's publications can be found on his Web site: www.yapko.com. Dr. Yapko is a member of the American Psychological

Association, a clinical member of the American Association for Marriage and Family Therapy, a member of the International Society of Hypnosis, and a fellow of the American Society of Clinical Hypnosis. He is a recipient of the Milton H. Erickson Award of Scientific Excellence for Writing in Hypnosis, and the 2003 Pierre Janet Award for Clinical Excellence from the International Society of Hypnosis, a lifetime achievement award honoring his many contributions to the field of hypnosis. He also received the Milton H. Erickson Foundation *Lifetime Achievement Award for Outstanding Contributions to the Field of Psychotherapy*.

Index